THE COMPLETE MRCPsych PART II

THE COMPLETE MRCPsych PART II

A comprehensive guide to the examination

Edited by Ashok G Patel MBBS, DPM, FRCPsych
Consultant in General Adult Psychiatry
Bedford Hospital
Bedford, UK

Hodder Arnold

A MEMBER OF THE HODDER HEADLINE GROUP

First published in Great Britain in 2006 by
Hodder Arnold, an imprint of Hodder Education and a member of the Hodder Headline Group,
338 Euston Road, London NW1 3BH

http://www.hoddereducation.com

Distributed in the United States of America by
Oxford University Press Inc.,
198 Madison Avenue, New York, NY 10016
Oxford is a registered trademark of Oxford University Press

Whilst the advice and information in this book are believed to be true and accurate at the date of
going to press, neither the author[s] nor the publisher can accept any legal responsibility or
liability for any errors or omissions that may be made. In particular, (but without limiting the
generality of the preceding disclaimer) every effort has been made to check drug dosages; however
it is still possible that errors have been missed. Furthermore, dosage schedules are constantly being
revised and new side-effects recognized. For these reasons the reader is strongly urged to consult
the drug companies' printed instructions before administering any of the drugs recommended in
this book.

British Library Cataloguing in Publication Data
A catalogue record for this book is available from the British Library

Library of Congress Cataloging-in-Publication Data
A catalog record for this book is available from the Library of Congress

ISBN-10   0 340 908 106
ISBN-13   978 0 340 908 105

1 2 3 4 5 6 7 8 9 10

Commissioning Editor: Clare Christian
Project Editor: Clare Patterson
Production Controller: Jane Lawrence
Cover Design: Nichola Smith
Index: Laurence Errington

Typeset in 9.5 on 12pt Rotis serif by Phoenix Photosetting, Chatham, Kent
Printed and bound in Malta

What do you think about this book? Or any other Hodder Arnold title?
Please send your comments to www.hoddereducation.com

CONTENTS

Section 3: Critical review paper

Section 4: Essay paper

Section 5: Individual patient assessment (IPA)

Section 6: Patient management problems (PMPs)

CONTRIBUTORS

Ashok G Patel MBBS, DPM, FRCPsych
Consultant in General Adult Psychiatry
Bedford Hospital
Bedford
UK

Elizabeth Barron MBChB, MRCPsych
Specialist Registrar to Dr Ashok G Patel
Bedford Hospital, Weller Wing
Bedford
UK

Sanjith Kamath MBBS, MRCPsych
Specialist Registrar
Broadfields Hospital
Cambridge
UK

Milind Karale MBBS, DPM, DNB, MRCPsych
Specialist Registrar
Adrian House
Fulbourn Hospital
Cambridge
UK

Vishelle Ramkisson MBBS, MRCPsych
Specialist Registrar
Lucille Van Geest Centre,
Peterborough District Hospital
Peterborough
UK

Simmi Sachdeva-Mohan MBBS, DPM, MD, MRCPsych
Specialist Registrar
Rampton Hospital
Nottingham Healthcare NHS Trust
Retford
Nottingham
UK

Kallol Sain MBBS, DPM, MRCPsych
Specialist Registrar
Old Age Psychiatry
Fulbourn Hospital
Cambridge
UK

Kirti Singh MBBS, PGDLMS
Senior House Officer in Accident and Emergency Medicine
Luton and Dunstable Hospital
Luton
Bedfordshire
UK

Ajay Upadhyaya DPM, MD, FRCP (Canada), FRCPsych
Consultant Psychiatrist
Herts and Essex Hospital
Bishop's Stortford
UK

FOREWORD

This is a thoroughly good book that I have enjoyed, immensely. Had I been a candidate for the MRCPsych Part II, I am sure that I would have come to rely on it during my preparation, seeing it as a guide and mentor, pointing me to other resources when necessary, and helping me to see both the wood and the trees. Together with its Part I companion, *The Complete MRCPsych Part II* will surely become a routine workbook for those intending to become Members of the Royal College of Psychiatrists. Well-thumbed copies will become treasured possessions, too familiar to give away once the examination is passed, but top of the list of recommendations for the next ranks of trainees. Books like this become friends.

This is, indeed, a comprehensive guide. The College examination has undergone considerable development and refinement over recent years, teaching as well as testing those who aspire to become modern psychiatrists. *The Complete MRCPsych Part II* begins by offering a comprehensive guide to the curriculum and the examination, showing candidates why these hurdles are before them. There is also a useful, general study guide. The following sections concentrate in turn on the new ISQ and EMQ formats, the Critical Reviews, the all too often neglected Essay paper, and the clinically orientated IPA and PMP sections. All formats are carefully explained such that no candidate need feel in the dark as to exactly what is required of them on the day.

An experienced, committed and sought-after clinical teacher, Dr Ashok Patel has brought together contributions from those who either match his expertise or who have the benefit of recent trials with the examination, a vital hybrid. The breadth and depth of the material exactly matches what is required. The format, with practice papers and model answers for each of the components, has a refreshing frankness: there are only three things necessary to perform well in anything, not just the MRCPsych examination: practice, practice and more practice. *The Complete MRCPsych Part II* will structure that practice, making sure that the basics become second nature (even statistics!) and that the details are familiar enough to allow candidates to sparkle.

As Dr Patel points out, this book is not just for trainees. Anyone with responsibilities for basic psychiatric training or who is involved with helping young psychiatrists through our College examination will find the book of use. I shall certainly keep a copy to hand, and recommend it to colleagues at any stage of their careers; all will take much from its pages.

Peter B. Jones
Professor of Psychiatry
University of Cambridge

PREFACE

This book is the product of many years' experience of clinical psychiatry and teaching both undergraduate and postgraduate students in psychiatry. It should serve as a framework to prepare for all topics of the different components of the MRCPsych Part II examination. It should also serve as a tool to test the knowledge of candidates taking this examination. The book is primarily aimed at senior house officers and other doctors (both referred to as candidates throughout the book). However, college tutors, coordinating tutors, specialist registrars and consultant psychiatrists/educational supervisors will also find it helpful in teaching and training their colleagues for the examination. I believe that the book will allow readers to become familiar with both the format and content of the examination, leading to success in the actual examination.

As the title of the book suggests, I have tried to cover all aspects of the curriculum for the examination. The book contains six papers of Individual Statement Questions (ISQs) with answers and explanations where necessary, and two papers of Extended Matching Items (EMIs) questions with answers. More importantly, guidance is provided on how to prepare for the examination, i.e. from the time of decision to take the examination until the day of taking it, and how to tackle it on the actual day. The ISQ papers contain a range of questions arranged in the manner as they appear in examination under headings. Candidates will therefore be able to concentrate their minds better, rather than when going through questions that are arranged randomly.

For the essay paper, critical review paper, individual patient assessment and patient management problems, there is information on how to prepare for the examination and how to tackle these on the day of the examination. This will help candidates to manage their time before and during the examination.

Throughout the book, my purpose has been to provide sufficient information for each component of the curriculum rather than a full account. It is therefore assumed that candidates will read textbooks and other publications before and while attempting the sample questions for obtaining more information. I have tried my best to give accurate answers and explanations to the ISQs and answers to the EMIs. However, it is possible that inaccuracy may have crept in. I would therefore advise readers to refer to textbooks and other authentic sources of information to verify the answers if necessary.

The Further Reading section includes a carefully selected list of books and other publications following advice from college tutors and trainees who passed this examination in recent years. As this is meant to be a guide to the examination, references for every statement are not provided. The candidates are advised to refer to the Further Reading section and other sources for relevant references if required.

I would like to thank the other contributors who volunteered to participate in the production of this book. I would like to thank the trainees who helped me to peer review the ISQs and EMIs and hopefully improve their quality. My sincere thanks to Professor Peter Jones for his most helpful encouragement, advice and his generosity in providing a Foreword. I am most grateful to the staff of Hodder Arnold, especially Clare Christian, Clare Patterson, and Lotika Singha for their advice and support throughout the preparations of the book.

It would not have been possible to produce this work without the support of our families.

A G P

SECTION 1:
A GUIDE TO THE MRCPsych PART II EXAMINATION

1 FORMAT OF THE MRCPSYCH PART II EXAMINATION AND FUTURE CONSIDERATIONS

There is no limit to the number of times a candidate can take the MRCPsych Part II Examination. The written examination has three parts:

- two multiple choice question papers
- one critical review paper
- one essay paper.

There is no negative marking in the written examination. The clinical examination has two parts:

- individual patient assessment
- patient management problems.

The written examination

Multiple choice question papers

One multiple choice question paper has questions from the **basic sciences** and the other covers **clinical topics**. Both papers consist of 165 Individual Statement Questions (ISQs) and 15 Extended Matching Items (EMIs) based on five themes. Each EMI has four components: the theme, options, lead-in (i.e. instructions) and three questions. See Section 2, Chapter 5 for further details of the format of these papers.

Time

A total of 90 minutes is allotted for each of the above papers. Candidates are advised to spend 75 minutes on the ISQs and 15 minutes on the EMIs.

Marking system

The total marks for each multiple choice question paper is 210, of which 165 marks are for the ISQs and 45 are for the EMIs. See Section 2, Chapter 5 for further details about the marking of EMIs.

For both papers, the marks in the ISQ and EMI sections are combined and converted to a closed score which will be between 0 and 10. The closed scores of both papers are then combined to give a total closed score.

Critical review paper

The critical review paper has two questions: A and B. In Question A, the candidate has to answer seven questions about the findings of a published paper. In Question B, the candidate will need to answer three questions on a short published research study, which is usually related to the study in Question A. The questions are based on the practice of evidence-based medicine (EBM). See Section 3, Chapter 16 for further details of the format of the critical review paper.

Time

A total of 90 minutes is allotted for the critical review paper.

Marking system

The whole paper carries a total of 100 marks, of which Question A is allotted 70 marks and Question B is allotted 30 marks. See Section 3, Chapter 16 for the further break down of the marks for both questions.

Essay paper

Candidates are required to answer ONE out of the three questions in the paper. Each question will encompass aspects of general adult psychiatry and one or more of the different psychiatric specialties. See Section 4, Chapter 20 for further details of the format of the essay paper.

Time

A total of 90 minutes is allotted for the essay paper.

Grading system

The essays are marked (graded) on a scale from 0 to 10 as follows:

0–1 = Very poor
2–3 = Fail
4 = Borderline fail
5 = Borderline pass
6–7 = Pass
8–10 = Excellent

The clinical examination

Individual patient assessment (IPA)

In the IPA examination the candidate is asked to examine a patient following which the candidate is interviewed by two examiners. See Section 5, Chapter 24 for further details of the format of the IPA.

Time

Candidates are allowed 60 minutes to examine the patient. The interview with the examiner lasts 30 minutes. Chapter 24 gives further details of the break down of the time the examiners will spend on examining various aspects of the IPA.

Marking system

A candidate's performance is marked on a scale from 0 to 10, with 5 as the pass mark.

Patient management problems (PMPs)

This part of the examination is also known as the Structured Oral Examination. Each candidate will be presented with three vignettes and all candidates taking the examination on the same day will be examined against the same vignettes. See Section 6, Chapter 28 for details of the format of the PMPs.

Time

The time allotted for PMPs is 30 minutes.

Marking system

A candidate's performance is marked on a scale from 0 to 10, with 5 as the pass mark.

Future considerations

The MRCPsych examinations are being continuously assessed and refined. With the establishment of the Postgraduate Medical Education and Training Board (PMETB), significant changes may be made to the format of written papers, especially the ISQ and EMI components. It is also possible that the format of the clinical examination may be changed, especially the long case, i.e. the IPA in Part II, to determine more precisely the interaction between the candidate and patient.

It is highly probable that progress through the training programme will be determined by competency-based assessments. The direction of change is difficult to predict at present, but it may include modularization of courses with assessment at the end of each module. The MRCPsych examinations will still be required as evidence of competencies acquired at the end of each training course. Major alterations may be made to the content of the present MRCPsych examinations, but the format will not necessarily change to the same extent.

2 OUTLINE OF THE CURRENT CURRICULUM

The following outline is meant to be a quick checklist only. Candidates should refer to the Royal College of Psychiatrists Council Report CR95 (*CR95. Curriculum for basic specialist training and the MRCPsych examination*, 2001) for more information.

Basic sciences

Psychology
- Basic, social, behavioural and neuropsychology
- Psychological assessment and psychometrics

Human development
- Preconceptual and prenatal influences on development
- Maturational process and ageing

Psychopathology
- Descriptive and dynamic psychopathology

Psychopharmacology
- General principles of prescribing, classification, pharmacogenetics, pharmacokinetics, pharmacodynamics, adverse drug reactions, and drug interactions
- Methodology of randomized controlled drug trials including design, randomization, blindness, statistical power, duration, rating scales and exclusion criteria

Social sciences
- Historical sociological theories of Weber, Marx, Durkheim, Foucault, Parsons, Gofman and Habermas
- Systems of social stratification slavery, castes, estate, class and theories of stratification (Marx, Weber)
- Social causes of illness and how life events, social support and social networks affect them, e.g. concepts of adversity and resilience, buffering, expressed emotion and their role in psychopathology
- Effects of sex and gender differences, stereotyping social roles, patriarchy, domestic violence, sexual harassment, racism, racial harassment, refugee status and impact of migration

- Relationship between culture, society and mental disorders, e.g. ethnicity, race, religion, attitudes, values and pluralist models of society
- History and philosophy of psychiatry

Neurosciences

- Neuroanatomy
  - General anatomy and functions of lobes and major gyri, prefrontal cortex, cingulate gyrus, limbic system, cranial nerves, spinal cord, basal ganglia, hippocampus and amygdala
  - Major white matter and neurochemical pathways
- Neuropathology
  - Organic brain disorders including dementias, head injuries, strokes, multiple sclerosis
  - Schizophrenia, conditions associated with mental retardation including autism
  - Movement disorders, e.g. Parkinson's disease, Huntington's disease and tardive dyskinesia
- Neurophysiology and neuroendocrinology
  - Physiology and anatomical pathways of the neural and endocrine systems
  - Hypothalamic and pituitary hormones involved in integrated behaviour such as perception, pain, memory, motor function, arousal, drives (sexual behaviour, hunger, thirst), motivation, and emotions including fear, aggression and stress
  - Physiology of neurones, synapses, and receptors including synthesis, release and uptake of neurotransmitters, action and resting potential, ion fluxes and channels
    Sleep, normal electroencephalogram (EEG) and evoked response techniques and their clinical applications
- Neurochemistry
  - Neurotransmitter synthesis, storage and release of noradrenaline, serotonin (5-hydroxytryptamine), γ-aminobutyric acid (GABA), acetylcholine, and excitatory amino acids
  - Functions of ion channels
  - Neuropeptides, in particular, corticotrophin releasing hormone, cholecystokinin and the encephalins/endorphins/dynorphins

Genetics

- Chromosomes, cell division, gene structure, transcription and translation
- Structure of human genome and patterns of inheritance
- Family, twin and adoption studies
- Molecular genetics, e.g. restriction enzymes, molecular cloning and gene probes, Southern blotting, restriction fragment length polymorphisms and recombination
- Prenatal identification and genetic counselling, DNA banks
- Molecular and genetic heterogeneity and phenotype/genotype correspondence

- Direct gene analysis and gene tracking including genetic markers, linkage studies and LOD (log of odds) scores

Epidemiology

- Basic concepts and measures in epidemiology: populations, samples, incidence, prevalence and risk, measures of association between cases, disease and exposure surveys, case–control studies, cohort studies and randomized control trials
- Epidemiological data, methods of sampling and how to interpret associations, procedure of screening for a particular disease in a population

Ethics and the law

- Legal principles, consent, restraint, legal responsibilities and protection
- Power of Attorney, Enduring Power of Attorney, living wills, management of assets and testamentary capacity
- Effects of mental disorders on driving capability

Critical appraisal skills

- Critical appraisal of a published scientific paper
- Study designs to test the hypothesis proposed in a paper
- Concepts used in evidence-based medicine, e.g. specificity, sensitivity, positive and negative predictive values, likelihood ratios, absolute and relative rate reduction, number needed to treat and odds ratios
- Common sources of bias, randomized controlled trials, cohort, case–control and single-case studies, economic analysis and qualitative study research
- Sampling, confidence intervals, probability and correlation coefficients, parametric tests (*t* tests, analysis of variance, multiple regression, etc.) and non-parametric tests (chi square test, Mann–Whitney U test, etc.)
- Systematic reviews and meta-analyses

Clinical topics

Mental disorders

- Major dimensions, classification and diagnosis
- Assessment including risk and management
- Preventive strategies

Gender issues and psychosexual disorders

- Disorders exclusive to women, e.g. postnatal depression, puerperal psychosis and premenstrual dysphoric disorder
- Disorders of sexual orientation and identity

Mental health services

- Service planning, development and management
- Multi-agency working

Psychiatry in relation to neurology and medicine

Child and adolescent psychiatry

- Epidemiology, clinical features, aetiology and management of mental disorders in childhood and adolescence
- Legal, ethical and structural framework underpinning child and adolescent mental health services
- Risk, vulnerability, resilience, and continuities and discontinuities throughout the life cycle

Learning disability

- Aetiology and development of learning disability
- Classification and epidemiology of mental disorders in learning disability
- Assessment and management of people with learning disability
- Provision of services

Liaison psychiatry

- Basic and clinical science as applied to problems seen in a general hospital
- Assessment and management of common mental disorders encountered in a general hospital
- Legal issues: current mental health legislation, common law, assessment of capacity to consent to or to refuse medical treatment

Forensic psychiatry

- Relationship between mental disorder and antisocial behaviour
- Principles of clinical risk assessment and management
- Relationships between psychiatry and the criminal justice system and the prison service
- Role of the psychiatrist in court
- Range of forensic psychiatric facilities and treatment

Old age psychiatry

- Clinical features, epidemiology and aetiology of the common mental disorders
- Principles and context of treatment of the common mental disorders
- Legal, ethical and structural framework underpinning old age psychiatry services
- Mental health legislation, Court of Protection, Enduring Power of Attorney, advocacy, living wills

Addiction psychiatry

- Main diagnostic categories: the World Health Organization International Classification of Diseases (ICD)-10 and the American Psychiatric Association Diagnostic and Statistical Manual (DSM)-IV
- Various models available for explaining the addictions
- Epidemiology of addictive disorders and psychiatric morbidity with addiction
- General principles and context of treatment, legal, ethical and structural framework underpinning the management of addiction-related disorders

Social and rehabilitation psychiatry

- Historical perspective and theoretical background, e.g. the 'pyramid of care' concept, the significance of care pathways, the interface between generic community mental health teams and specialist rehabilitation services
- Range of tertiary rehabilitation services, e.g. supported and residential accommodation

Psychotherapy

- Psychological development at all stages of the life cycle
- Main contributors to psychoanalytic theories: Sigmund Freud, Jung, Klein, Winnicott, Kohut, Kernberg, Balint, Erikson, Fairburn, Harman, Bion and Anna Freud
- Principles and practice of:
  - Cognitive–behavioural therapy
  - Behaviour modification and social skills training
  - Psychoanalytic psychotherapy
  - Short-term dynamic, brief focal therapies, interpersonal therapy, and cognitive analytic therapy
  - Group psychotherapy, therapeutic communities
  - Family therapy

Perinatal psychiatry

- Epidemiology, clinical features, aetiology and management of common mental disorders occurring in perinatal period

Transcultural psychiatry

- Influence of race, culture and religion on psychiatry
- Epidemiology, clinical presentation, course and outcome of major mental disorders across cultures

3 HOW TO PREPARE FOR THE EXAMINATION

The MRCPsych II Examination is a test of knowledge and skills, and requires a great deal of hard work and preparation. Papers such as the critical review paper and the basic sciences multiple choice question paper require an intimate understanding of the facts and processes that many junior doctors do not routinely use in their daily clinical practice. In preparing for the MRCPsych examination, a vast quantity of information has to be understood and facts memorized, ready to be regurgitated in a trice in the examination hall.

There is no shortage of guidebooks and psychiatric texts available. It is hard for any candidate not to feel overwhelmed by the amount of reading that passing the examination appears to necessitate. However, like most examinations, passing the MRCPsych II involves reading the right things from the right books and a complex interplay between hard work and luck. What prospective candidates can try to do is minimize the extent to which luck controls the outcome of their performance in the examination.

When should one start preparing for the examination?

The answer to this question obviously depends on individual ability and competence. Although many examiners will tell candidates that they should start studying for the examination at the time they start training, in the real world this is not practical. Anyone who has a family and a busy on-call rota will know how difficult it is get any sort of studying done unless there is a strong motivation to do so, such as an examination around the corner. As a rule of thumb, it is often recommended that the best time to start studying is around **6 months** prior to the examination. This will coincide with the announcement of the results of the written paper of the previous examination, and this should sufficiently motivate prospective candidates.

Studying for the examination

Timetable

The first thing to do is to make a timetable for the next six months on each day of the week. Candidates should give themselves a break every 4–5 days.

Months 1–3

Candidates should amass material from various sources:

- Try to obtain individual statement questions (ISQs), extended matching item (EMIs) questions and notes from colleagues who have passed the examination
- Buy/borrow textbooks (see Further reading at the end of the book)
- Check out websites on the internet (see links below)

Start by reading textbooks on general psychiatry, concentrating on 'big' topics such as affective disorders and schizophrenia initially and then moving on to other topics including the specialties. The idea behind this is to ease oneself into studying by starting off with things that everyone is (hopefully!) more familiar with. Candidates should start reading for the basic sciences paper in much the same way, beginning with topics they are more familiar with (from the MRCPsych I, for example). They should aim to finish one small topic a day of each (general psychiatry and basic sciences) and allow two days for each large topic.

Practising with ISQ and EMI papers at this stage is likely to be demoralizing. Candidates should start flicking through a critical review textbook from page 1. Suppress the urge to look at the papers at the beginning of the revision. Unless one has a special interest in statistics or an aptitude for mathematics, attempting a critical review paper at this stage will frighten some candidates very badly.

Aim to finish reading the textbooks in the first three months. Candidates should not worry if they cannot remember most of what was read in this time. The idea is simply to familiarize oneself with terms and concepts. Therefore, spend the first two months reading textbooks on both clinical topics and the basic sciences and, as mentioned above, collecting information from websites and colleagues who have passed the examination. Make a list of tentative essay topics – again colleagues and a look through current journals for topical issues will be helpful.

Months 3–5

Now things start to get serious, and the candidate should now be in the habit of reading something every day. Also, from this point onwards, practise around 100 ISQs every day in addition to the reading. Keep track of the scores in a book. Most hard working candidates are pleasantly surprised by how their scores improve over the days in the next two months. The authors used to practise ISQs during on-calls, because it was not necessary to concentrate too much on memorizing and interruptions were not too disruptive.

As well as the above, candidates should work on the critical review paper for an hour each day. The idea here is to get used to focusing the mind on different types of problems over a few hours (like in the examination). Prepare two essay plans each week (over the weekend for example).

By the end of the fifth month some 6000 ISQs and several EMIs should have been done and 16 essay plans prepared. In addition, candidates would have worked for approximately 60 hours on the critical review paper.

Month 6

Crunch time!

The authors recommend that candidates apply for at least two weeks' leave before the written papers. Even more if it can be managed! If candidates cannot get study leave, they should consider taking annual leave or even leave without pay. It may seem like a big sacrifice but it will be worth it. If candidates plan their timetable right, they will be able to apply for leave well in advance. This is important, especially if the job demands locum cover, which will need to be arranged. Nearer the time of the examination, consider swapping on-calls so that they can be done after the examination.

In month 6, candidates should continue revising from textbooks, reading relevant journals (e.g. *British Journal of Psychiatry*, and *Advances in Psychiatric Treatment*), practising ISQs and EMIs, preparing essay plans and answering critical review papers according to their individual requirements every day.

Practise writing quickly and neatly. Try to finish the critical review paper in less than the allocated time. If candidates feel less confident about a topic, they should try to go through an examination guidebook quickly spending not more than half an hour on it.

By the last month, between 6000 and 10 000 ISQs and a few hundred EMIs (of which many will be repeat questions) should have been done, about 30 essay plans prepared and about 30 critical review papers answered.

Which courses should one attend?

There is no clear-cut answer to this question. There are people who have passed without attending a single course (except the mandatory day release course), but again there are people who have been unsuccessful despite attending numerous courses.

Most courses are useful because they help to focus the candidate's attention on what is important and current. Courses also give the candidates a chance to compare themselves with other candidates, which is an important psychological factor in determining how they are doing. One of the most useful aspects of any course is the hand-outs, which includes notes, ISQs and EMIs. However, bear in mind that most courses go over the same things so it is important not to waste time listening to the same things again. Therefore, the authors suggest the following guide to attending courses that should be of adequate help for preparation for the examination.

- Attend a course six months before the exam (for example, the Guildford course; see www.guildfordcourse.co.uk). This will give candidates an idea of what they need to study and which areas of the curriculum need relatively more attention.

- Attend a critical review course a month or two before the examination. Remember that this will be a revision course so it is essential that candidates should have completed at least one reading of the critical review books before they attend otherwise the time and money spent on this course would not be worth it.
- Attend a revision course one month before the course (for example, the Manchester course; see www.manchestercourse.com). This will help the candidates to focus on the most recent developments, the likely essay topics and help with the final preparations for the examination.

Places on most courses are limited so the candidates should book a place as early as possible.

Helpful hints

- One should keep a topic-wise list of references for the essays in a book and guard it with one's life.
- Reading journals can be time consuming but try to read the last 12 issues of *Advances in Psychiatric Treatment*. It really helps in preparing the essay plans.
- Don't spend too much time on any one ISQ or EMI. Some people spend hours trying to find the right answer with the right reference. It's just not worth the time and effort. Candidates should remember they are working to a tight schedule.
- Make a list of things that are 'volatile', i.e. difficult to remember. This will largely be a subjective list but may include neuroanatomy facts, critical review definitions, formulae, etc. Go over these topics again and again.
- Study in groups if it helps, but candidates should not let other people slow them down. This is not the time to be 'carrying' people.
- Stay calm during the examination as nothing messes with one's memory like anxiety.

Pitfalls

- Starting too early: The aim is to be at the peak at the right time, i.e. the exam day. Studying too hard too early can lead to burnout.
- Starting too late: Pretty obvious but some people do make this mistake. There is no substitute for hard work.
- Reading too much into an ISQ or EMI: some of them are phrased ambiguously and a lot of people wonder whether the College is trying to 'trick' them. Remember the College is not trying to trick anyone, so second guessing isn't helpful.
- Writing a wonderful essay but not on the given topic. Read the question carefully and stick to addressing only the relevant issues.

This chapter was about some of the things that helped the authors and their friends with the examination. The authors are aware that they may not be the only or the best methods in the world but the methods worked for them. Above everything else, remember that one can pass this examination – with a bit of luck and a lot of hard work.

Further reading

http://www.superego-cafe.com

SECTION 2:
INDIVIDUAL STATEMENT QUESTIONS (ISQs) AND EXTENDED MATCHING ITEMS (EMIs)

4 OUTLINE OF THE CONTENTS OF THE ISQ AND EMI PAPERS

Individual Statement Questions (ISQs) and Extended Matching Items (EMIs) were introduced in both the basic sciences and clinical topics written papers for the MRCPsych Part II in autumn 2003. The breakdown of ISQs in the papers in this book (as suggested by the Royal College of Psychiatrists) is a rough guide, intended to give candidates an idea of the areas of the curriculum that are covered by the examination. However, questions on other areas of the curriculum may be included. The exact number of questions from each area is also a rough guide. There is no official breakdown that covers the EMI component of either the basic sciences or the clinical topics paper. In both papers:

- ISQs = 165
- EMIs = 5, each containing three questions (=15 questions)

Breakdown of ISQs

Basic sciences paper

Psychology – 62 questions

Basic and behavioural	9
Social	12
Neuropsychology	14
Human development	17
Assessment	5
Description and measurement of behaviour	3
Basis of psychological treatments	2

Social sciences and ethology – 14 questions

Neurosciences – 39 questions

Neuroanatomy	5
Neuropathology	9
Neurophysiology	10
Neuroendocrinology	8
Neurochemistry	7

Psychopharmacology (pharmacokinetics, pharmacodynamics, adverse drug reactions, theories of action, drug dependence, new drugs) – 18 questions

Genetics, epidemiology, statistics and research methodology, medical ethics and principles of law – 32 questions

Clinical topics paper

General adult psychiatry (classification of disease, preventive strategies, presentation of illness and treatment, hospital liaison psychiatry, neuropsychiatry, medicine relevant to psychiatry and HIV, research) – 56 questions

Old age psychiatry – 25 questions

Addictions – 17 questions

Child and adolescent psychiatry – 24 questions

Forensic psychiatry – 16 questions

Learning disability – 19 questions

Psychotherapy and psychopathology – 8 questions

5 FORMAT OF THE ISQ AND EMI PAPERS

Individual Statement Questions

Format

Individual Statement Questions (ISQs) are single-stem statements with no relation to any of the other statements. However, there may be two or three consecutive statements on the same theme. Candidates are advised to consider each question on its own merit and answer as true or false. As stated in Chapter 1 there is no negative marking.

Extended Matching Items

Format

There are four elements in the structure of an Extended Matching Item (EMI):

- Theme: This is a short title that focuses the candidate's attention on the subject of the question. For example, 'Management of depression'. It should help candidates to focus on a single, clear issue. The title will, therefore, encompass both the skills* and the knowledge** to be tested.
- Option list: This is a list of possible answers to the questions that follow, for example the list may give a number of treatment options or diagnoses or clinical features. The list will be based on only one area of skill/knowledge and will NOT contain a mix of different areas, for example, diagnosis and treatment. The option list is therefore a homogeneous mix of items.
- Instructions (lead-in): This part tells the candidates about the task that has to be carried out.
- Questions: These are the problems which have to be solved by selecting the correct answers from the option list. Under each theme there are three questions.

*Skills: These include a variety of areas such as diagnostic skills, procedural skills, communication, bedside manner, etc.

**Knowledge: This covers the information acquired during the training period, for example, mood disorders, anxiety disorders, schizophrenia.

Reasons for the introduction of EMIs

The idea behind EMIs is to minimize the recognition effect that tends to occur in standard multiple choice question papers. This is achieved by the many possible combinations of vignettes and options. By using clinical cases instead of facts, the items can be used to test application of knowledge and problem-solving ability.

EMIs are easier to construct than key feature questions, as many questions can be drawn from one set of options, and the reliability has been shown to be good. EMIs are best when large numbers of similar kinds of decision, for example, relating to diagnosis or ordering of laboratory test needs to be tested for different situations. EMIs are more likely to test clinical reasoning, that is, the application of clinical knowledge to practical situations.

The disadvantage of EMIs is that there is a risk of under-representation of certain themes simply because they do not fit the format of the test.

Skills and knowledge to be tested

- Diagnosis/differential diagnosis
- Clinical and procedural skills
- Investigations/selection and interpretation of diagnostic tests
- Management

Context of clinical management

- Decisions supported by evidence including the principles of risk management, involving patients and, where appropriate, their relatives or carers in decisions about their care.
- Good practice in prescribing.
- Effective communication skills including listening, questioning, explaining, involving patients in management, sharing information, recognizing that patients are knowledgeable, discussing options with patients and explaining the effects of treatment and procedures.
- Awareness and sensitivity of the need and expectations of patients regardless of their lifestyle, culture, beliefs, ethnicity, gender, sexuality, disability, age or social or economic status and understanding the patient's environment and its effects on their health.
- Disease factors such as inherited diseases and the natural history of disease.
- Practice of evidence-based medicine.
- Understanding of epidemiological principles and prevalence of important diseases in the UK.
- Awareness of methods of prevention and health promotion.
- Application of current scientific basis/understanding of mental disorders.
- Awareness of the different attitudes/behaviour that may be encountered in a multicultural society and appreciation of the impact of sociocultural factors on the incidence and prevalence of mental disorders.

Marking of EMIs

There are two types of EMI:

- R type, i.e. single best answer (3 marks)
- N type, i.e. multiple best answers
  - Two best answers (1.5 marks for each correct answer, total 3 marks)
  - Three best answers (1 mark for each correct answer, total 3 marks)

In questions with two and three best answers, only the first two and three answers, respectively, will be scored and the rest of the answers will be ignored.

6 HOW TO PREPARE FOR AND TACKLE ISQ AND EMI PAPERS

Preparing for ISQs and EMIs

Candidates should review the core curriculum carefully and revise topics according to the number of questions per topic. For example, there are more questions from general adult psychiatry in the clinical topics paper; hence more attention should be paid to this topic. There is no substitute for extensive revision. A number of sources of ISQs and EMIs are available, including this book.

How to tackle ISQs

Candidates should give appropriate weight to each part of the paper according to the number of questions from each theme. Some candidates are good at psychology or dynamic psychopathology whereas others might find these topics relatively more difficult. Hence, all candidates are advised to identify their weaknesses by practising answering sample papers and taking part in group revision well before the actual examination.

How to tackle EMIs

Consider the range of topics in the section on 'Skills and knowledge to be tested' in Chapter 5. Candidates should read the question first and then look for the answer(s) in the options list. Remember that the theme, i.e. the main area of the skills and knowledge being tested, informs what the EMI is about e.g. diagnosis, investigations. This should help candidates to concentrate on the given exercise.

Remember that the questions require the best answer(s). Usually the number of correct answers for each question will be as required by the question. However, there may be other correct answers but which may not necessarily be the best answers. The majority of the EMIs will require the candidate to choose one best answer, but a few will require two to three answers for each question.

7 TERMS USED IN THE ISQ AND EMI PAPERS

Occurs	Does not give any indication of frequency of occurrence
Usually	60% or more
Recognized	Means it has been reported to occur as a feature or association
Characteristic	Features that occur often enough so as to be of some diagnostic value and whose absence might lead to doubts about the diagnosis
Diagnostic, essential and typical features	Must occur to make a diagnosis
Specific or pathognomonic	Features that occur in the named disease and no other
Can be or may be	Features are reported as occurring
Commonly, frequently, is likely or often	All imply a rate of occurrence greater than 50%
Particularly associated	Implies a significant association in some samples with sufficient numbers
Implicit	Implied although not plainly expressed
Explicit	Expressly stated
Exclusively	Features that occur in the named condition and no other
Invariably	Implies the occurrence of a feature without a shadow of doubt
Includes	Similar to 'occurs', i.e. makes no mention of frequency
Majority	More than 50%

8 BASIC SCIENCES: PAPER 1 (ISQs)

Sample questions

Psychology

Basic, behavioural and social psychology

1   Cognitive dissonance is a concept originally developed by social psychologists.

2   Cognitive dissonance is usually found in patients suffering from social phobia.

3   Cognitive dissonance is usually found in patients with bipolar affective disorder.

4   Cognitive dissonance makes up for low self-esteem.

5   Cognitive dissonance is a cause of internal discomfort in human beings.

6   Conditioned avoidance is a manifestation of neurotic anxiety, which can lead to reinforcement of conditioned emotional response.

7   Conditioned avoidance is a manifestation of neurotic anxiety, which can lead to discrimination of conditioned stimuli.

8   Conditioned avoidance is a manifestation of neurotic anxiety, which can lead to elimination of operant behaviour.

9   Conditioned avoidance is a manifestation of neurotic anxiety, which can lead to superstitious behaviour.

10 Conditioned avoidance is a manifestation of neurotic anxiety, which can lead to diminution of the strength of the conditioned response.

11 The process of generalization of the conditioned stimulus strengthens instrumental responses.

12 Instrumental responses are strengthened by the process of acquisition of autonomic emotional responses.

13 The process of elimination of negative and conditioned stimuli strengthens instrumental responses.

14 The process of trial and error strengthens instrumental responses.

15   The process of reinforcement of the required voluntary behaviour strengthens instrumental responses.

[Answers on page 48]

Neuropsychology

16   Visuospatial difficulties are a characteristic feature of parietal lobe lesions.

17   Topographic disorientation is a characteristic feature of parietal lobe lesions.

18   Anosognosia is a characteristic feature of parietal lobe lesions.

19   Gerstmann's syndrome is a manifestation of parietal lobe lesions.

20   Agraphaesthesia is a characteristic feature of parietal lobe lesions.

21   Motor aphasia is a characteristic feature of dominant temporal lobe lesions.

22   Severe amnesic syndrome is a characteristic feature of dominant temporal lobe lesions.

23   Alexia is a feature of dominant temporal lobe lesions.

24   Agraphia is a characteristic feature of dominant temporal lobe lesions.

25   Constructional apraxia is a characteristic feature of dominant temporal lobe lesions.

[Answers on page 48]

Human development

26   The language developmental milestone of counting up to 10 is normally achieved by 3 years of age.

27   The language developmental milestone of uttering three or more words is achieved by 18 months of age.

28   The language developmental milestone of giving his or her name is achieved by 30 months of age.

29   The language developmental milestone of use of 'mama' and 'dada' is generally achieved by 1 year of age.

30   The language developmental milestone of use of sentences of up to four words is normally achieved by 2.5 years of age.

31   According to Piaget's theory, circular reaction is a part of the preoperational stage of human development.

32   According to Piaget's theory, the law of conservation is a part of the preoperational stage of human development.

33   According to Piaget's theory, precausal reasoning is a part of the preoperational stage of human development.

34   According to Piaget's theory, phenomenalistic causality is a part of the preoperational stage of human development.

35   According to Piaget's theory, animistic thinking is a part of the preoperational stage of human development.

36   Crawling or toddling to the mother is a characteristic feature of attachment behaviour.

37   Using the mother as a secure base from which to explore the surroundings is a characteristic feature of attachment behaviour.

38   Clinging hard when anxious is a characteristic feature of attachment behaviour.

39   Crying frequently in the mother's presence is a characteristic feature of attachment behaviour.

40   Climbing onto the mother's lap, having not seen her for a while, is a characteristic feature of attachment behaviour.

[Answers on page 48]

Assessment, description and measurement of behaviour

41   According to psychoanalytic theory, projective identification is one of the mental mechanisms involved in dreams.

42   According to psychoanalytic theory, projection is one of the mental mechanisms involved in dreams.

43   According to psychoanalytic theory, secondary revision is one of the mental mechanisms involved in dreams.

44   According to psychoanalytic theory, desymbolization is one of the mental mechanisms involved in dreams.

45   According to psychoanalytic theory, dissociation is one of the mental mechanisms involved in dreams.

46   Most psychoanalysts would agree that anal eroticism leads to sodomy.

47   Most psychoanalysts would agree that anal eroticism leads to homosexuality.

48   Most psychoanalysts would agree that anal eroticism leads to miserliness.

49   Most psychoanalysts would agree that anal eroticism leads to bestiality.

50   Most psychoanalysts would agree that anal eroticism leads to obsessional states.

51   Denial is a narcissistic defence mechanism of the ego.

52   Primitive idealization is a narcissistic defence mechanism of the ego.

53   Projective identification is a narcissistic defence mechanism of the ego.

54   Rationalization is a narcissistic defence mechanism of the ego.

55   Reaction formation is a narcissistic defence mechanism of the ego.

56   According to the psychoanalytic theory of development of personality, genetic factors play a minimal role.

57   According to the psychoanalytic theory of development of personality, it is completed within the first 7 years of life.

58   According to the psychoanalytic theory of the development of personality, the Oedipus complex occurs in the phallic phase.

59   According to the psychoanalytic theory of the development of personality, parental guidance is usually considered important in the development of the child.

60   According to the psychoanalytic theory of the development of personality, mentally impaired patients have delayed development of their personality.

61   A psychometric assessment of personality can be made with the Present State Examination (PSE).

62   A psychometric assessment of personality can be made with the Montgomery–Åsberg Depression Rating Scale.

63   The Thematic Apperception Test can be used to assess personality.

64   A psychometric assessment of personality can be made by using the Sentence Completion Test.

65   A psychometric analysis of personality can be made with the Repertory Grid Test.

[Answers on page 49]

Basis of psychological treatments

66   According to psychoanalytic theory, condensation is a mental mechanism involved in dreams.

67   According to psychoanalytic theory, symbolism is a mental mechanism involved in dreams.

68   According to psychoanalytic theory, sublimation is a mental mechanism involved in dreams.

69   According to psychoanalytic theory, rationalization is a mental mechanism involved in dreams.

70   According to psychoanalytic theory, displacement is a mental mechanism involved in dreams.

71   Semantic differentials are essentially described as 'forced choice' techniques.

72   Semantic differentials are commonly used to measure qualitative aspects of attitudes.

73   Semantic differentials are most useful in differentiating schizophrenic thought disorder from non-schizophrenic thought disorder processes.

74   Semantic differentials involve the use of unipolar adjectival pairs.

75   Semantic differentials are not contaminated with a tendency to evoke social desirability in the respondents.

76   From the viewpoint of psychoanalysis, if children are given adequate sex education most neurotic disorders can be prevented.

77   From the viewpoint of psychoanalysis, the roots of most adult neurotic problems can be traced to sexual seduction in childhood.

78   From the viewpoint of psychoanalysis, negativism is an early warning feature of adolescent crisis.

79   From the viewpoint of psychoanalysis, the mother–child relationship during the first year of life is an important factor in determining the child's psychological development.

80   From the viewpoint of psychoanalysis, counter-transference is essential for a successful outcome of the therapy.

81   The General Health Questionnaire is an observer-rated psychometric instrument.

82   Leyton Obsessional Inventory is an observer-rated psychometric instrument.

83   Severity of Alcohol Dependence Questionnaire (SADQ) is an observer-rated psychometric instrument.

84   Present State Examination is an observer-rated psychometric instrument.

85   Beck's Depression Inventory is an observer-rated psychometric instrument.

[Answers on page 50]

Social sciences and ethology

86   Eye to eye contact is usually determined by cultural factors.

87   Eye to eye contact is one of the essential ingredients of analytical psychotherapy.

88   Eye to eye contact is influenced by hormonal changes.

89   Eye to eye contact is reduced in Alzheimer's disease.

90   Eye to eye contact remains unaffected in depressed patients.

91   With regard to styles of leadership, members of a group with an autocratic leader are aggressive towards one another.

92   With regard to styles of leadership, democratic leaders yield greater productivity.

93   With regard to styles of leadership, the laissez-faire leadership style is good for urgent problems.

94   With regard to styles of leadership, members of a group with a democratic leader abandon their task in the leader's absence.

95   With regard to styles of leadership, the laissez-faire style is good for creative and original results.

96   According to the New York longitudinal study, the dimensions of behaviour of young children include persistence.

97   According to the New York longitudinal study, the dimensions of behaviour of young children include aggression.

98   According to the New York longitudinal study, the dimensions of behaviour of young children include quality of mood.

99   According to the New York longitudinal study, the dimensions of behaviour of young children include distractibility.

100   According to the New York longitudinal study, the dimensions of behaviour of young children include obstinacy.

101   As regards social classes, social class III has the highest mortality for men aged 15–64 years.

102   Social class I has the lowest mortality due to tuberculosis.

103   Social class V has the highest mortality due to chronic bronchitis.

104   Social class V has the highest rates of chronic illnesses for both men and women.

105   Social class V has the fewest number of visits to general practitioners.

106   Imprinting is a form of social attachment seen in various species.

107   Imprinting is known to occur in primates.

108   Imprinting occurs during the first few months of life.

109   In imprinting, anticipatory anxiety is a common feature.

110   Imprinting may be related to unacceptable sexual impulses.

[Answers on page 50]

Neurosciences

Neuroanatomy

111   Fornix is a part of the limbic system.

112   The limbic system includes the amygdaloid complex of nuclei.

113   Olfactory bulbs form part of the limbic system.

114   The limbic system includes the striae terminalis.

115   Olive is a part of the limbic system.

116   The neuroglia include interstitial cells that completely fill the gaps between the nerves.

117   The number of neuroglia is almost twice the number of neurones in the brain.

118   Neuroglia are mesodermal in origin.

119   Neuroglia form part of the blood–brain barrier.

120   Neuroglia are usually involved in the synthesis of neurotransmitters in the brain.

121   Posterior spinocerebellar tract is an ascending white matter tract of the spinal cord.

122   Fasciculus cuneatus is an ascending white matter tract of the spinal cord.

123   Tectospinal tract is an ascending white matter tract of the spinal cord.

124   Lateral corticospinal tract is an ascending white matter tract of the spinal cord.

125   Lateral spinothalamic tract is an ascending white matter tract of the spinal cord.

126   Blood supply to the optic radiation is provided by the anterior communicating artery.

127   Central branches of the anterior cerebral artery provide blood supply to the optic radiation.

128   Posterolateral branches of posterior cerebral artery provide blood supply to the optic radiation.

129 Blood supply to the optic radiation is provided by the anterior choroidal artery.

130 The posterior cerebral artery provides blood supply to the optic radiation.

131 Occlusion of the dominant middle cerebral artery at its origin causes contralateral exaggerated deep reflexes.

132 Occlusion of the dominant middle cerebral artery at its origin causes difficulty in understanding both written and spoken speech.

133 Occlusion of the dominant middle cerebral artery at its origin causes contralateral hemiplegia.

134 Occlusion of the dominant middle cerebral artery at its origin causes positive Babinski's sign.

135 Occlusion of the dominant middle cerebral artery at its origin causes partial ipsilateral facial weakness.

136 Significant memory impairment is caused by lesions in the hippocampus.

137 Lesions in Broca's area cause significant memory impairment.

138 Lesions in mamillary bodies cause significant memory impairment.

139 Significant memory impairment is caused by lesions in the fornix.

140 Lesions in anterior perforated substance cause significant memory impairment.

141 Loss of conscious proprioception is a characteristic feature of posterior column lesions.

142 Loss of pain sensation is a characteristic feature of posterior column lesions.

143 Loss of touch discrimination is a characteristic feature of posterior column lesions.

144 Loss of sensation of body image is a characteristic feature of posterior column lesions.

145 Cerebellar ataxia is a characteristic feature of posterior column lesions.

146 Purkinje cells send axons to cerebellar nuclei.

147 Purkinje cells receive direct innervations from mossy fibres.

148 Purkinje cells contain gamma-aminobutyric acid (GABA) in high concentration.

149 Purkinje cells characteristically degenerate in Pierre-Marie's hereditary cerebellar ataxia.

150 Purkinje cells send efferents to the lateral vestibular nucleus.

151 With reference to the cerebral cortex in human beings, the neocortex constitutes about 90 per cent of the cerebral cortex.

152 The cerebral cortex in humans consists of six cellular layers.

153 The cerebral cortex in humans consists of 17 Brodmann's areas.

154 The cerebral cortex in humans is a sheet of white matter.

155 The cerebral cortex in humans contains Martinotti's cells.

156 A neurocyte is part of a neurone.

157 A nucleus is part of a neurone.

158 The neuroglia is part of a neurone.

159 The myelin sheath is part of a neurone.

160 Synaptic cleft is part of a neurone.

[Answers on page 51]

Neuropathology

161 Primary demyelination occurs in Huntington's disease.

162 Primary demyelination occurs in Parkinson's disease.

163 Primary demyelination occurs in the Wernicke–Korsakoff syndrome.

164 Primary demyelination occurs in Krabbe's disease.

165 Primary demyelination occurs in the Marchiafava–Bignami disease.

166 The prion dementias characteristically show spongy degeneration of the cerebral grey matter.

167 The prion dementias characteristically show neuronal proliferation.

168 The prion dementias characteristically show amyloid protein identical to that seen in Alzheimer's disease.

169 The prion dementias characteristically show astrocytic proliferation.

170 The prion dementias characteristically show Lewy bodies in the brain stem.

171 Neuritic plaques are characteristic pathological features of dementia in Alzheimer's disease type 2.

172 Reactive astrocytosis is a characteristic pathological feature of dementia in Alzheimer's disease type 2.

173 Hirano bodies are characteristic pathological features of dementia in Alzheimer's disease type 2.

174 Lewy bodies are characteristic pathological features of dementia in Alzheimer's disease type 2.

175 Amyloid angiopathy is a characteristic feature of dementia in Alzheimer's disease type 2.

176 Neuritic plaques are characteristic features of Alzheimer's disease.

177 The number of neuritic plaques correlates with the degree of intellectual decline.

178 Neuritic plaques are a characteristic feature of dementia pugilistica.

179 Neuritic plaques are a diagnostic feature of punch-drunk syndrome.

180 Neuritic plaques are intracellular brain structures.

181 Nissl substance is composed of rough endoplasmic reticulum.

182 Nissl substance appears as coarse granules under a light microscope.

183 Nissl substance synthesizes protein for the nervous system.

184 Nissl substance is a component of lysosomes.

185 Nissl substance may be found in white blood cells.

[Answers on page 53]

Neurophysiology

186 An abnormal brain respiratory rate is found in Alzheimer's disease.

187 An abnormal brain respiratory rate is found in catatonic stupor.

188 An abnormal brain respiratory rate is found in depressive stupor.

189 An abnormal brain respiratory rate is found in Huntington's disease.

190 An abnormal brain respiratory rate is found in generalized anxiety disorder.

191 Biofeedback is a system that involves administration of a reward and punishment to neurotic patients.

192 Biofeedback is an effective method of modifying cardiovascular functions.

193 Biofeedback involves the provision of information to the patients.

194 Biofeedback is a useful method of conditioning the involuntary autonomic nervous system.

195   Biofeedback teaches the patient to regulate some of the physiological functions.

196   Carbamazepine causes fast activity on the electroencephalogram.

197   Chlorpromazine causes fast activity on the electroencephalogram.

198   Fluoxetine causes fast activity on the electroencephalogram.

199   Lithium carbonate causes fast activity on the electroencephalogram.

200   EEG changes after a course of electroconvulsive therapy usually persist for about a week.

201   The serum prolactin level rises shortly after electroconvulsive therapy.

202   The plasma cortisol level falls within an hour of the electroconvulsive therapy.

203   After electroconvulsive therapy, there is an initial period of bradycardia followed by tachycardia.

204   After electroconvulsive therapy, there is a decrease in cerebral circulation.

205   An abnormal electroencephalogram is commonly found in patients with subdural haematoma.

206   An abnormal electroencephalogram is commonly found in patients with narcolepsy.

207   An abnormal electroencephalogram is commonly found in patients suffering from night terrors.

208   An abnormal electroencephalogram is commonly found in patients with antisocial personality disorder.

209   An abnormal electroencephalogram is commonly found in patients with a cerebral abscess.

210   Penile erection occurs in rapid eye movement (REM) sleep.

211   Penile erection is impaired in patients with severe depression.

212   Penile erection is exaggerated in patients with generalized anxiety disorder.

213   Anticholinergic agents decrease penile erection.

214   Penile erection is facilitated by the sacral roots of parasympathetic nerves.

215   Starvation leads to increased levels of endorphin in the cerebrospinal fluid (CSF) in patients with anorexia nervosa.

216   Vivid dreams are a recognized feature of REM sleep.

217   Nightmares are a recognized feature of REM sleep.

218   Loss of muscle tone is a recognized feature of REM sleep.

219   Increased alpha activity in the electroencephalogram (EEG) is a recognized feature of REM sleep.

220   Biochemical effects of electroconvulsive therapy include a sudden rise of noradrenaline.

221   Biochemical effects of electroconvulsive therapy include a sudden rise in the plasma concentration of 5- hydroxyindoleacetic acid (5-HIAA).

222   Biochemical effects of electroconvulsive therapy include a rise in prolactin levels.

223   Biochemical effects of electroconvulsive therapy include a reduction in plasma levels of adrenocorticotrophin-releasing hormone (ACTH).

224   Plausible explanations of the therapeutic effects of electroconvulsive therapy include a reduction in the plasma concentration of noradrenaline.

225   Plausible explanations of the therapeutic effects of electroconvulsive therapy include a decrease in dopamine function.

226   Plausible explanations of the therapeutic effects of electroconvulsive therapy include an increase in 5-hydroxytryptamine (5-HT) function.

227   Plausible explanations of the therapeutic effects of electroconvulsive therapy include an increase of corticotrophin releasing hormone (CRH) concentration in cerebrospinal fluid.

228   Plausible explanations of the therapeutic effects of electroconvulsive therapy include a blunting of thyroid stimulating hormone (TSH) response to thyrotrophin-releasing factor.

229   As regards electroconvulsive therapy, the magnitude of the electrical stimulus has a strong relationship to its untoward effects.

230   As regards electroconvulsive therapy, the magnitude of the electric stimulus has a strong relationship to seizure threshold.

231   As regards electroconvulsive therapy, the seizure time has a strong relationship to its efficacy.

232   Seizure threshold rises and seizure duration shortens during the course of a typical series of electroconvulsive treatments.

233   As regards electroconvulsive therapy, memory impairment is associated with the amount of electrical stimulus.

234 Unilateral electroconvulsive therapy to the dominant cerebral hemisphere appears to induce less memory impairment than bilateral treatment.

235 Memory impairment following a course of six sessions of electroconvulsive therapy usually resolves within 3 months.

[Answers on page 54]

Neuroendocrinology

236 Somatostatin facilitates the release of glucagons from the pancreas.

237 The cortical concentration of somatostatin is diminished in patients with Alzheimer's disease.

238 Bombesin is functionally related to kinesin.

239 Bombesin is a potent appetite stimulant.

240 Bombesin stimulates the release of prolactin and growth hormone.

[Answers on page 55]

Neurochemistry

241 The selective serotonin reuptake inhibitor drugs are extensively eliminated by hepatic metabolism in the form of mostly inactive metabolites.

242 Norfluoxetine is an active metabolite of fluoxetine.

243 Fluoxetine has a shorter half-life than other similar compounds that are currently available.

244 The washout period of fluoxetine is over several weeks.

245 The selective serotonin reuptake inhibitor drugs have clinically insignificant cardiotoxic effects in overdoses.

246 As regards neurotransmitters, the precursor of dopamine is an amino acid with an aromatic side chain.

247 The precursor of noradrenaline is an amino acid with a basic side chain.

248 Tryptophan is the precursor of serotonin.

249 Glycine has an aliphatic side chain.

250 Glutamate is an amino acid with a basic side chain.

251 Phosphoinositide pathway is a second messenger pathway.

252 Phosphoinositide pathway is triggered by the enzymatic clearance of phosphatidylinositol biphosphate.

253   In the phosphoinositide pathway, the active second messengers are inositol triphosphate (IP3) and inositol tetraphosphate (IP4).

254   In the phosphoinositide pathway, the compounds inositol triphosphate (IP3) and inositol tetraphosphate (IP4) stimulate a rise in intracellular sodium.

255   The phosphoinositide pathway may explain the mechanism of action of lithium carbonate.

256   The clinical effects of stimulation of dopamine receptors include sedation.

257   The clinical effects of stimulation of dopamine receptors include nausea and vomiting.

258   The clinical effects of stimulation of dopamine receptors include diuresis.

259   The clinical effects of stimulation of dopamine receptors include dyskinesias.

260   The clinical effects of stimulation of dopamine receptors include drive.

261   Acetylcholine is a principal neurotransmitter in presynaptic sympathetic ganglia.

262   Acetylcholine is a principal neurotransmitter in the spinal Renshaw cells.

263   Acetylcholine is a principal neurotransmitter in presynaptic parasympathetic ganglia.

264   Acetylcholine is a principal neurotransmitter in the mesolimbic tract.

265   Acetylcholine is a principal neurotransmitter in the neuromuscular junction.

266   G-protein coupled receptors have seven transmembrane spanning sites.

267   G-protein coupled receptors have five intracellular loops.

268   G-protein coupled receptors have an extracellular C-terminal.

269   G-protein coupled receptors have an intracellular N-terminal.

270   G-protein-coupled receptors belong to several distinct super families of central nervous system receptors.

271   According to current scientific knowledge, the inotropic receptors are part of the super family of G-protein coupled receptors.

272   According to current scientific knowledge, inotropic receptors include N-methyl-D-aspartate (NMDA) receptors.

273 According to current scientific knowledge, inotropic receptors contain a central ion channel.

274 According to current scientific knowledge, inotropic receptors involve charged particles (ions), which pass through the ionophore to enter the neurone.

275 According to current scientific knowledge, stimulation of inotropic receptors causes rapid changes in neuronal excitability.

276 According to current scientific knowledge, memantine is a glutamatergic modulator for the treatment of Alzheimer's disease.

277 According to current scientific knowledge, glutamate is the most prevalent excitatory neurotransmitter in the brain.

278 According to current scientific knowledge, glutamate is central to approximately 80 per cent of the systems associated with cognition and memory.

279 Memantine blocks pathological activation of N-methyl-D-aspartate (NMDA) receptors by excessive glutamate, while preserving physiological function.

280 Memantine restores synaptic signal detection and synaptic plasticity allowing learning and memory function.

[Answers on page 56]

Psychopharmacology

Pharmacokinetics

281 The serum level of carbamazepine may be increased by concomitant administration of cimetidine.

282 The serum level of carbamazepine may be decreased by concomitant administration of other anticonvulsant drugs.

283 The serum level of carbamazepine may be increased by concomitant administration of verapamil.

284 Carbamazepine metabolism in the body may be decreased by concomitant administration of tricyclic antidepressant drugs.

285 Carbamazepine metabolism may be increased by concomitant administration of antipsychotic drugs.

286 Patients with adjustment disorders usually show a marked non–drug-specific response and/or sustained spontaneous recovery.

287 Patients with dissociative states usually show a marked non–drug-specific response and/or sustained spontaneous recovery.

288   Patients with drug-induced psychosis usually show a marked non–drug-specific response and/or sustained spontaneous recovery.

289   Major depressive episodes usually show a marked non–drug-specific response and/or sustained spontaneous recovery.

290   Manic episodes usually show a marked non–drug-specific (placebo) response and/or sustained spontaneous recovery.

291   With regard to the effects of drugs on human performance, assessment of sensory function is by the critical flicker fusion (CFF) threshold.

292   With regard to the effects of drugs on human performance, paper and pencil tests, such as digit symbol substitution measure central nervous system arousal.

293   According to current scientific knowledge, prolonged treatment with non-selective monoamine oxidase inhibitors (MAOIs) results in 'downregulation' of 5-hydroxytryptamine 2 (5-HT$_2$) receptors.

294   According to current scientific knowledge, the non-selective monoamine oxidase inhibitors markedly reduce rapid eye movement (REM) sleep.

295   Non-selective monoamine oxidase inhibitors are highly water soluble.

296   Monoamine oxidase inhibitors are mainly excreted unchanged by the kidneys.

297   As regards the pharmacokinetics of monoamine oxidase inhibitors, the acetylation status is polygenically inherited.

298   According to current scientific knowledge, tricyclic antidepressant drugs inhibit the reuptake of noradrenaline and 5-HT into the nerve terminals.

299   According to current scientific knowledge, the antimuscarinic action of tricyclic antidepressant drugs is the basis of many of their peripheral side effects.

300   According to current scientific knowledge, tricyclic antidepressant drugs have a little affinity for alpha-2 adrenoreceptors.

301   According to current scientific knowledge, prolonged treatment with tricyclic antidepressant drugs leads to 'downregulation' of beta adrenoreceptors.

302   According to current scientific knowledge, long term treatment with tricyclic antidepressant drugs leads to a decrease in the number of D$_2$ receptors.

303   According to current scientific knowledge, tricyclic antidepressant drugs increase awakenings during sleep.

304   According to current scientific knowledge, tricyclic antidepressant drugs decrease the latency to the onset of REM sleep.

305   According to current scientific knowledge, tricyclic antidepressant drugs reduce the REM sleep duration.

306   Tricyclic antidepressant drugs are lipid soluble.

[Answers on page 57]

Pharmacodynamics

307   As regards pharmacodynamic interactions, phenothiazines potentiate the central depressant actions of antihistaminic drugs.

308   Phenothiazines decrease the analgesic effects of opiates.

309   Phenothiazines potentiate the central depressant effect of general anaesthetics.

310   Butyrophenones cause a marked increase in intracellular lithium.

311   Antipsychotic drugs enhance the dopaminergic effects of antimuscarinic drugs.

312   According to current scientific knowledge, tolerance to the antipsychotic effect of haloperidol does not occur.

313   According to current scientific knowledge, tolerance to the antipsychotic effect of chlorpromazine does not occur.

[Answers on page 58]

Adverse drug reactions

314   An abstinence syndrome is known to be caused by prolonged administration of zopiclone.

315   Prolonged administration of buspirone is known to cause an abstinence syndrome.

316   An abstinence syndrome is known to be caused by prolonged use of caffeine.

317   An abstinence syndrome is known to be caused by prolonged administration of methaqualone.

318   Prolonged administration of paroxetine is known to cause an abstinence syndrome.

319   Carbamazepine has a three-ringed structure similar to the tricyclic antidepressant drugs.

320   The commonest side effects of carbamazepine are due to raised plasma concentration.

321   An allergic rash is a rare side effect of carbamazepine.

322   Hepatotoxicity is a common side effect of carbamazepine.

323   Carbamazepine is frequently fatal in overdose.

[Answers on page 58]

Genetics

324   An X linked inheritance is ruled out if affected fathers have affected sons.

325   In recessive inheritance, where both parents are known to be carriers, there is a 25 per cent chance that each child will be affected.

326   In autosomal dominant inheritance, each child of an affected parent has a 50 per cent chance of developing the condition.

327   As regards mode of inheritance, a similar prevalence of a particular disorder in both siblings and off springs of an index case strongly supports the probability of an autosomal dominant inheritance.

328   In polygenic inheritance, environmental factors have no role to play.

329   Coffin–Lowry syndrome occurs only in females.

330   Glucose-6-phosphate dehydrogenase deficiency occurs only in females.

331   Aicardi's syndrome occurs only in females.

332   Niemann–Pick disease occurs only in females.

333   Rett's syndrome occurs only in females.

334   Cri-du-chat syndrome is transmitted by a single dominant gene.

335   Acute intermittent porphyria is transmitted by a single dominant gene.

336   Rett's syndrome is transmitted by a single dominant gene.

337   Acrocallosal syndrome is transmitted by a single dominant gene.

338   Acrodysostosis is transmitted by a single dominant gene.

339   Current scientific knowledge suggests that Huntington's disease is transmitted by a single dominant gene.

340   Current scientific knowledge suggests that schizophrenia is transmitted by a single dominant gene.

341   Current scientific knowledge suggests that Alpert's syndrome is transmitted by a single dominant gene.

342   Current scientific knowledge suggests that phenylketonuria is transmitted by a single dominant gene.

343   Current scientific knowledge suggests that Creutzfeldt–Jakob disease is transmitted by a single dominant gene.

344   Attention deficit and hyperactivity are recognized features of fragile X syndrome.

345   Female carriers of fragile X syndrome are less impaired than male fragile X carriers.

346   A small head and ears and small stature are characteristic features of fragile X syndrome.

347   Tall stature is a recognized feature of fragile X syndrome.

348   Postpubertal macro-orchidism is a recognized feature of fragile X syndrome.

349   Down's syndrome is the most commonly studied cause of learning disability.

350   Down's syndrome is associated with an increased risk of bipolar affective disorder in the affected individuals.

351   Down's syndrome is associated with an increased risk of further affected children in young mothers with translocation chromosome.

352   Down's syndrome may be caused by increased age of the father.

353   Down's syndrome is associated with symptomatic carriers who have only 45 chromosomes.

[Answers on page 58]

Epidemiology

354   Interviewing a patient's relatives is an essential feature of a prospective epidemiological study.

355   A longitudinal follow-up is an essential feature of a prospective epidemiological study.

356   Random allocation of patients to treatment groups is an essential feature of a prospective epidemiological study.

357   Use of existing case controls is an essential element of a prospective epidemiological study.

358   Psychiatric case registers are essential in prospective epidemiological studies.

359   Epidemiological studies include population surveys.

360   Epidemiological studies include double blind clinical trials.

361   Epidemiological studies include cohort studies.

362   Epidemiological studies include use of case registers.

363   Epidemiological studies include use of hospital morbidity rates.

[Answers on page 59]

Statistics and research methodology

364   The Yerkes–Dodson curve demonstrates the relation between the level of arousal and the efficiency of performance.

365   The Yerkes–Dodson curve is an inverted U-shaped curve.

366   The Yerkes–Dodson curve is modified by high levels of anxiety.

367   The Yerkes–Dodson curve is primarily concerned with drive and performance.

368   The Yerkes–Dodson curve is unaffected by alterations in the level of consciousness.

369   Placebo washout for a short period is important in assessing the effectiveness of a new drug treatment.

370   Constrained randomization is important in assessing the effectiveness of a new drug treatment.

371   Subjective rating scales are important in assessing the effectiveness of a new drug treatment.

372   The placebo control group is important when assessing the effectiveness of a new drug treatment.

373   Crossover design is important in assessing the effectiveness of a new drug treatment.

374   The standard deviation is a statistical measure of statistical significance.

375   The standard deviation is a statistical measure of frequency.

376   The standard deviation is a statistical measure of dispersion.

377   The standard deviation is a statistical measure of variance.

378   The standard deviation is a statistical measure of departure from the arithmetic mean.

379   Standard intelligence tests are of little value in people over the age of 65 years.

380   Standard intelligence tests can be modified to meet the special needs of a patient.

381   Standard intelligence tests usually yield normal distribution scores in a general population.

382   Standard intelligence tests can be used universally without any difficulties.

383   Standard intelligence tests are a most useful tool for differentiating multi-infarct dementia from other types of dementias.

384   Concerning the measurement of risk, a value of 1 for the relative risk implies a causal association.

385   Concerning the measurement of risk, the odds ratio is useful in prospective studies.

386   Concerning the measurement of risk, the attributable risk is also known as the risk difference.

387   Concerning the measurement of risk, the value of 0 for the attributable risk implies an association.

388   Concerning the measurement of risk, the odds ratio is an approximation of attributable risk.

389   All trials in a meta-analysis should satisfy minimum standards for random allocation of patients.

390   All trials in a meta-analysis should satisfy minimum standards for blind assessment.

391   All trials in a meta-analysis should satisfy minimum standards for measurements.

392   All trials in a meta-analysis should satisfy minimum standards for outcome criteria.

393   All trials in a meta-analysis should satisfy minimum standards for treatment variables.

[Answers on page 59]

Medical ethics and principles of law

394   Under no circumstances do the principles of beneficence and non-maleficence override the principle of respect for the patient's autonomy.

395   Under no circumstances, does the clinician have a duty to warn and protect third parties placed at risk by a patient without his or her knowledge and agreement.

396   The primacy of autonomy implies that a patient's competence to make choices about his/her treatment is a dichotomous either/or phenomenon.

397   The primacy of the contractarian model of the relationship between doctor and patient includes respect for a patient's autonomy.

398   Respecting a patient's autonomy assumes that a patient's mental capacity to make informed choices is not impaired temporarily or permanently by a mental or physical disorder.

399   In the teleological model of the doctor–patient relationship, the principles of non-maleficence and beneficence are fundamental.

400   In the therapeutic relationship between doctor and patient, the principle of justice does not require attention to means by which the benefits and burdens for compulsory treatment of a patient balance against those accrued to other people.

[Answers on page 60]

Answers

Psychology

Basic, behavioural and social psychology

1   True
2   False
3   False   This occurs when there is a palpable discrepancy between the experimental or behavioural elements. It is not confined to any specific diagnostic category.
4   True
5   True
6   True
7   True
8   False
9   True
10   False
11   False
12   False
13   False
14   True
15   True

Neuropsychology

16   True
17   True
18   True   Anosognosia refers to loss of awareness of neurological deficit.
19   True
20   True   Agraphaesthesia is the inability to name figures drawn on the hand.
21   False   This is caused by lesions in Broca's area.
22   False   This results from bilateral lesions of the medial temporal lobe structures.
23   True   Caused by posterior lesions of the temporal lobe.
24   False
25   False

Human development

26   False   The child can count up to 10 by age 4.
27   True
28   True
29   True
30   False   The child can use sentences of 4 words by age 3.
31   False   Circular reaction occurs in the sensorimotor stage.

32   **False**   Law of conservation is a part of the concrete operational stage of cognitive development.
33   **True**
34   **True**
35   **True**
36   **True**
37   **True**
38   **True**
39   **False**
40   **True**

Assessment, description and measurement of behaviour

41   **False**   Projective identification allows one to distance and make oneself understood by exerting pressure on another person to experience feeling similar to one's own.
42   **True**
43   **True**
44   **True**
45   **True**
46   **False**   Sodomy is anal intercourse.
47   **False**   Freud viewed homosexuality as an arrest in psychosexual development. He believed that female homosexuality was due to a lack of resolution of penis envy in association with unresolved Oedipal conflicts.
48   **True**
49   **False**   Bestiality is the use of an animal as a repeated and preferred or exclusive method of achieving sexual excitement.
50   **True**
51   **True**
52   **True**
53   **True**
54   **False**   It is a neurotic defence mechanism.
55   **False**   It is a neurotic defence mechanism.
56   **False**
57   **False**
58   **True**
59   **False**
60   **False**   According to psychoanalytic theory, our personalities are basically determined by inborn drives and environmental influences in the first 5 years.
61   **False**   It is useful in assessing symptoms of psychotic patients.
62   **False**   It is useful in rating the severity of depression.
63   **True**   It is a projective test.
64   **True**   It is a projective test.
65   **True**   It is useful in revealing the characteristics of neurotic patients.

Basis of psychological treatments

66   True
67   True
68   False   Sublimation of aggressive impulses takes place through pleasurable activity and sports.
69   False   Rationalization is a justification of attitudes, beliefs or behaviour that may otherwise be unacceptable by incorrect application of justifying reasons.
70   True
71   True
72   False
73   True
74   True
75   False
76   False
77   False
78   False   Mild anxiety, depression and disagreement with authority figures are early signs of adolescent crisis.
79   True
80   False   Countertransference can be an impediment but it can be turned into an advantage.
81   False   It is a self-rating scale.
82   False
83   False
84   True
85   False   It is a self-rating scale.

Social sciences and ethology

86   True
87   False
88   False
89   True
90   False   Downcast eyes with vertical furrows on the brow with a slight rising of the medial aspect of each eye.
91   True
92   True
93   False   An autocratic style of leadership is good for solving urgent problems.
94   False
95   True
96   True
97   False
98   True
99   True

100 False   A total of nine dimensions of behaviour were identified. In addition
to those mentioned in Questions 96, 98 and 99 these include activity levels,
rhythmicity of biological functions, and approach/withdrawal to novelty,
adaptability, threshold of responsiveness to stimuli and intensity of
reaction.
101 False
102 True
103 False
104 True
105 False   Social class studies reveal that those in class V have the highest
rates of disease and visit their general practitioners frequently.
106 True
107 False   There is no evidence that it occurs in primates.
108 True   This is a special form of learning, quite different from ordinary
conditioning. It is limited to a very brief period, is fixed soon after birth
and is irreversible.
109 True
110 False

Neurosciences

Neuroanatomy

111 True
112 True
113 True
114 True
115 False   Olive is a part of the medulla oblongata.
116 True
117 False   About 5–10 times the number of neurones.
118 False   Neuroglia are ectodermal in origin.
119 True
120 False
121 True
122 True
123 False
124 False
125 True
126 False
127 False
128 True
129 True
130 True
131 True   The overriding effect of damage to the upper motor neurones is a
withdrawal of inhibition from spinal reflexes resulting in hyperreflexia and
hypertonia.

132 **True** Wernicke's aphasia is a disorder of reception, which leads to impairment of comprehension of spoken language.

133 **True**

134 **True** When the superficial plantar reflex is abolished by an upper motor neuron lesion, Babinski's sign is unmasked.

135 **False**

136 **True**

137 **False** This area is associated with expressive speech.

138 **True** The other structures associated with memory include amygdala, uncus and the dorsomedial nucleus of the thalamus.

139 **True**

140 **False**

141 **True** Posterior columns (medial lemniscal pathways) convey conscious and discriminative touch.

142 **False**

143 **True**

144 **True** These columns provide the parietal lobes with instantaneous body image, so that we are constantly aware of our body parts, both at rest and during movements.

145 **False**

146 **False** Purkinje cell axons are only efferent fibres from the cerebellar cortex that travel to other parts of the brain.

147 **False** Like the climbing fibres, the terminal fibres of olivocerebellar tracts, mossy fibres are the terminal fibres of all other cerebellar afferent tracts. They do not send direct innervation to Purkinje cells.

148 **True** The inhibitory signals from the Purkinje cells contribute to the final output from the cerebellum.

149 **True** Pathologically, hereditary ataxia of Pierre-Marie is indistinguishable from other hereditary degenerations or Friedreich's ataxia.

150 **True** Other efferents are to the vestibule and reticular neurones and the thalamus.

151 **True**

152 **True**

153 **False** Brodmann distinguished 47 regions in the cerebral cortex on the basis of difference in their cellular architecture. Many of these were subsequently identified as functional units, including the motor cortex, premotor cortex, visual cortex, auditory cortex, somatosensory cortex, etc.

154 **False**

155 **True**

156 **True** A neurone or nerve cell consists of a cell body or soma, known as perikaryon or neurocyte and neurites the axons and dendrites.

157 **True** The other structures include the nucleolus, Nissl substance, Golgi apparatus, microfilaments, microtubules and lysosomes.

158 **False** Neuroglial cells, also known as interstitial cells, make up most of the nervous tissue, outnumbering neurones 5–10 times.

159 **False**   The axon of a neurone may be ensheathed in a lamellated, interrupted covering called the myelin sheath.

160 **False**   It is a gap at the junction of two neurones.

Neuropathology

161 **False**   There is neuronal loss in the cerebral cortex, particularly affecting the frontal lobes, and in the corpus striatum of the basal ganglia.

162 **False**   There is depigmentation and neuronal loss of substantia nigra, particularly of the zona compacta.

163 **False**   There is secondary demyelination due to severe deficiency of thiamine (Vitamin B_1).

164 **False**   Due to deficiency of the enzyme galactocerebroside-beta-galactosidase, this leads to secondary demyelination.

165 **False**   This is caused by chronic alcohol abuse. There is widespread demyelination in the brain.

166 **True**

167 **False**   Neurones cannot regenerate.

168 **False**   Prion dementias are represented by Creutzfeldt–Jakob disease, Gerstmann–Strüussler syndrome and kuru.

169 **True**

170 **False**   Lewy bodies in the cerebral cortex are characteristic of Lewy body dementia.

171 **True**   Alzheimer's disease type 2 is an early onset dementia i.e. before the age of 65. Neuritic or senile plaques are extracellular argyrophilic bodies, which also occur in normal elderly people.

172 **True**

173 **True**   They are small eosinophilic neuronal inclusion bodies.

174 **False**   They are part of the cortical pathology of dementias associated with Parkinson's disease.

175 **True**   This is deposition of amyloid around small blood vessels.

176 **True**   The major pathological changes in Alzheimer's disease include widespread cerebral atrophy, neuronal loss, neuritic plaques and neurofibrillary tangles.

177 **True**

178 **False**   See answer 179.

179 **False**   Histological changes include cortical neuronal loss and neurofibrillary degeneration with neurofibrillary tangles in the cortex and the brain stem. Neuritic plaques are not present.

180 **True**

181 **True**   The Nissl substance (chromatophilic substance) is characteristic of nerve cells.

182 **True**

183 **True**

184 **False** Lysosomes are spherical, membrane-bound bodies containing a number of powerful enzymes. They act as the neuronal digestive system or as internal scavengers.

185 **False**

Neurophysiology

186 **True**

187 **False**

188 **False**

189 **True**

190 **False**

191 **False**

192 **True**

193 **True**

194 **True**

195 **True** Biofeedback is the application of operant conditioning in which human subjects are given feedback on their autonomic nervous system functioning or motor function. They are taught to exert some control over these systems.

196 **True**

197 **False** It decreases beta (high frequency) activity and increases delta and/or theta (low frequency) activity.

198 **False** It increases delta (low frequency) activity.

199 **False** It produces insignificant electroencephalographic changes.

200 **False** Electroencephalogram changes consist of intermittent diffuse irregular delta (low frequency) activity, which increases after each treatment. The electroencephalogram returns to normal 3 months after the completion of treatment.

201 **True**

202 **False** Plasma cortisol levels are raised after a single treatment and the rise lasts for 2–4 hours.

203 **True** Changes in blood pressure mirror changes in pulse rate.

204 **False** Cerebral circulation increases dramatically during either spontaneous or electrically induced epileptic seizures. Electroconvulsive therapy produces a large increase in the permeability of the blood–brain barrier.

205 **True** Classically there is an asymmetry with reduced amplitude activity on the affected side but more often there is an increased localized irregular slow activity with sleep waves.

206 **False**

207 **False**

208 **True** The typical finding is that of generalized, widespread slow (theta) wave activity occurring in 31–58 per cent of people with antisocial personality disorder. The 'positive spike' phenomenon is found in 40–45 per cent of aggressive and impulsive types of patient.

209 **True**   Extremely slow focal delta waves are recorded.
210 **True**
211 **True**   This is associated with loss of libido.
212 **False**   Penile erection is generally unimpaired but generalized anxiety disorder may be associated with loss of libido and premature ejaculation.
213 **False**
214 **True**   The exact mechanism of penile erection is not completely understood. It is a consequence of stimulation of sacral parasympathetic fibres or sympathetic inhibition, which triggers the vascular response.
215 **True**
216 **True**
217 **True**
218 **True**
219 **False**   The electroencephalograhic pattern of REM sleep is similar to stage 1 of non-REM sleep, i.e. low frequency theta activity with superimposed saw-toothed waves. Within the sleeping time, the proportion of REM sleep to non-REM sleep diminishes from approximately 50 per cent in the full-term newborn baby to less than 20 per cent by middle age.
220 **True**
221 **False**
222 **True**   It is probably linked to stimulation of 5-hydroxytryptamine 1 (5-HT$_1$) receptor subtype.
223 **False**
224 **True**
225 **False**   An increase in dopamine function.
226 **True**
227 **False**   A decrease in CRH concentration in cerebrospinal fluid.
228 **False**   No blunting. Baseline thyrotropin n-releasing hormone (TRH) and TSH are unaffected by a course of electroconvulsive therapy.
229 **False**
230 **True**
231 **False**   Little relationship is there. Seizures less than 20 seconds are likely to be the result of inadequate stimulus in relation to a patient's seizure threshold.
232 **True**
233 **True**   Appears to be so, and also to the site of electrodes.
234 **False**   Non-dominant hemispheres.
235 **False**   After about 6 months.

Neuroendocrinology

236 **False**   Somatostatin suppresses glucagon release.
237 **True**
238 **False**   Kinesin is an ATPase that is structurally similar to myosin. It is involved in axonal transport.
239 **False**   It inhibits feeding and induces satiety. It is thermostatin.
240 **True**   It is also an antidiuretic.

Neurochemistry

241 **True**

242 **True**

243 **False**   After long-term administration, the elimination half-life of fluoxetine is about 8 days. The other compounds have a shorter half-life.

244 **True**   Norfluoxetine, an active metabolite, has an elimination half-life of about 20 days. A period of several weeks is required for the drug to be washed out. Caution is necessary when prescribing drugs that interact with fluoxetine.

245 **False**   Current knowledge suggests that these compounds have clinically and pharmacologically insignificant cardiotoxic effects in therapeutic doses. They have some cardiotoxic effects in overdose, but are usually not fatal.

246 **True**

247 **False**

248 **True**

249 **True**

250 **False**

251 **True**   It is linked to a number of membrane-bound receptors through an intermediate G-protein.

252 **True**

253 **True**

254 **False**   The activation leads to an increase in intracellular calcium.

255 **True**

256 **False**

257 **True**

258 **False**

259 **False**   Depletion of dopamine leads to Parkinson's disease and possibly other movement disorders.

260 **True**   Dopamine release promotes drive reinforcement and an experience of pleasure.

261 **True**   Acetylcholine is the primary excitatory transmitter at the neuromuscular junction and preganglionic autonomic nerves.

262 **False**

263 **True**

264 **False**   Dopamine is the principal neurotransmitter involved with the mesolimbic tract.

265 **True**   There are two distinct types of acetylcholine receptor: nicotinic, which gate sodium channels, and muscarinic, which are linked to the G-proteins and phosphoinositol cycle.

266 **True**

267 **False**   They have three intracellular loops.

268 **False**   They have an extracellular N-terminal.

269 **False**   They have an intracellular C-terminal.

270 **False**   The G-protein receptors form one of the super families of central nervous system receptors. A super family consists of receptors that share several common features.

271 **False**   These receptors form one of the super families of brain receptors.

272 **True**   Ionotropic receptors also include nicotinic, cholinergic, gamma-aminobutyric acid A (GABA$_A$) and kainate receptors.

273 **True**

274 **True**

275 **True**   Because of the rapid changes in neuronal excitability that occur when these receptors are stimulated, the drugs acting on these receptors have a narrow therapeutic window.

276 **True**

277 **True**

278 **True**

279 **True**

280 **True**

Psychopharmacology

Pharmacokinetics

281 **True**

282 **True**

283 **True**

284 **False**

285 **True**

286 **True**

287 **True**

288 **True**

289 **True**

290 **True**

291 **False**   CFF exploits the phenomenon that a decrease in the arousal of the central nervous system (CNS) is accompanied by a fall in the maximum frequency of a light that can be detected.

292 **False**   This assesses sensory function, recognition or perception.

293 **True**   Also 5-HT$_A$ receptors.

294 **True**   There is a rebound increase in REM sleep on discontinuation of treatment.

295 **False**   Highly lipid soluble rapidly absorbed and widely distributed.

296 **False**   Extensively metabolized by liver. Only 1–2 per cent is excreted unchanged in the urine.

297 **False**   They have a monogenically inherited acetylation status.

298 **True**

299 **True**

300 **True**

301 **True**   Also 5-HT$_2$

302 **False** D_1 receptors are decreased. $GABA_B$ receptors are increased.
303 **False** They decrease awakenings during sleep.
304 **False** They increase it.
305 **True**
306 **True** They are rapidly and widely distributed in the body. They cross plasma and the blood–brain barrier.

Pharmacodynamics

307 **True** They also enhance the effects of alcohol and benzodiazepines.
308 **False** They increase the analgesic effects of opiates.
309 **True** They also potentiate the hypotensive effects of general anaesthetic drugs.
310 **False** They cause a minor decrease in intracellular lithium.
311 **False** Antipsychotic drugs antagonize the dopaminergic effects of antimuscarinic drugs.
312 **True**
313 **True** But tolerance develops to the sedative effect.

Adverse drug reactions

314 **True**
315 **True** There are anecdotal reports of withdrawal symptoms after short administration of zopiclone and buspirone. However, there is a strong suspicion that an abstinence syndrome may occur following prolonged administration.
316 **True**
317 **True**
318 **True**
319 **True**
320 **True**
321 **False** It consists of raised red, patchy skin lesions, which occur in 12–15 per cent of psychiatrically ill patients treated with carbamazepine.
322 **False** Rare side effect.
323 **False** Fatal overdose is rare.

Genetics

324 **True** In X linked inheritance, male to male transmission does not occur.
325 **True** 1 in 4 children are affected.
326 **True**
327 **True**
328 **False** Environmental factors have an important role to play in various types of inheritance, including polygenic inheritance.
329 **False** It is an X-linked disorder and affects males and females in equal numbers. Symptoms are more severe in males.
330 **False**
331 **True** Very rare in XXY genotype male.

332 False
333 True   It is an X-linked disorder. Male fetuses with the defective X chromosome are usually aborted. Cases have been reported in boys with XXY genotype and mosaicism.
334 False   It is caused by partial deletion of the short arm of chromosome 5.
335 True   It is also known as porphobilinogen deaminase deficiency or the Swedish type of porphyria.
336 True   Mutation on X chromosome presenting with characteristic deterioration of hand skills and stereotyped hand movements.
337 False   It is characterized by absence of corpus callosum, macrocephaly and severe learning disability. Autosomal recessive on chromosome 12.
338 True   It is characterized by alopecia, psychomotor epilepsy, pyorrhoea and learning disability.
339 True   Autosomal dominant disorder.
340 False   Schizophrenia does not seem to follow Mendel's laws of inheritance.
341 True   Autosomal dominant disorder.
342 False   Autosomal recessive disorder.
343 False   It does not seem to follow Mendel's laws of inheritance.
344 True
345 True
346 False   Usually large head and ears.
347 False   Short stature.
348 True
349 True
350 False
351 True
352 True
353 True   Relatives have an increased risk of Alzheimer's disease.

Epidemiology

354 False   Useful in retrospective studies
355 True
356 False
357 False   It is an element of retrospective studies.
358 True
359 True
360 False   Double blind clinical trials are designed to reduce bias in research studies.
361 True
362 True
363 True

Statistics and research methodology

364 True
365 True

366 True
367 True
368 False
369 True It is necessary to identify placebo responders and also patients whose illness responds spontaneously.
370 True It ensures that a number of patients are entered in similar proportions in each treatment group.
371 True
372 True It is one of the most important requirements during the initial assessment of a new drug.
373 False It is helpful in assessing treatment differences within the same subjects.
374 False Statistical significance is measured by tests like the *t* test.
375 False Frequency distribution is a systematic way of arranging data.
376 True
377 True Variance is a measure arrived at by squaring all the deviations, adding them up, and dividing the total by the number of measures.
378 True
379 False They are helpful in assessing older people.
380 True
381 True
382 False As they are in English, translations in other languages may not be accurate.
383 False
384 False The relative risk of a disease with respect to a given risk factor is the ratio of the incidence of the disease in people exposed to the incidence of the disease in the people not exposed. A value of 1 implies no causation.
385 False
386 True The attributable risk is the incidence of the disease in the group exposed to the risk factor minus the incidence in the group not exposed.
387 False A value of zero implies no association.
388 True
389 True
390 True
391 True
392 True
393 True

Medical ethics and principles of law

394 False If the patient is competent, his or her autonomy is paramount. However, if the patient is incompetent, breaches of confidentiality may be justified in his or her best interests. The principles of beneficence and non-maleficence override respect for the patient's autonomy.
395 False The General Medical Council says that such circumstances confer on doctors a duty of care to others.

396 **False**   Competence is task specific and not a global or dichotomous phenomenon.

397 **True**

398 **True**

399 **True**   Non-maleficence means to avoid harming those in the doctor's care and their kin. Beneficence means to do good or promote wellbeing.

400 **False**

9 BASIC SCIENCES: PAPER 2 (ISQs)

Sample questions

Psychology

Basic, behavioural and social psychology

1   Cognitive dissonance is a concept derived from social psychology.

2   Cognitive dissonance is a useful concept for cognitive–behavioural therapy.

3   Cognitive dissonance is usually not recognized by the subject.

4   Adding new cognition, which is consistent with the pre-existing ones, may reduce cognitive dissonance.

5   Cognitive dissonance has been used to analyse different patterns of smoking.

6   Operant conditioning may be understood in terms of perceptual expectancies.

7   Intermittent reinforcement in operant conditioning leads to greater resistance to extinction than with continuous reinforcement.

8   Punishment leads to diminished probability of the occurrence of a response.

9   Negative reinforcement is synonymous with punishment.

10   Extinction is the process of gradual disappearance of a conditioned response on discontinuation of an unconditional stimulus.

11   Classical conditioning takes place irrespective of the time interval between the conditioned stimulus and the unconditioned stimulus.

12   Classical conditioning takes place irrespective of the genetic potential of the organism.

13   Classical conditioning takes place irrespective of the organism's voluntary behaviour.

14   Classical conditioning takes place irrespective of the schedule of reinforcement.

15   Classical conditioning takes place irrespective of the nature of the unconditioned stimulus.

16   Research has demonstrated convincingly that females have relatively better visuospatial awareness than males.

17   Research has demonstrated convincingly that males excel in mathematical skills compared with females.

18   Research has demonstrated convincingly that females have relatively poorer verbal skills than males.

19   Research has demonstrated convincingly that males have relatively better non-verbal skills than females.

20   Research has demonstrated convincingly that females excel in passive aggression compared with males.

21   Classical conditioning occurs most effectively when the time intervals between the conditioned stimulus and the unconditioned stimulus are varied.

22   Classical conditioning occurs most efficiently when the unconditioned stimulus precedes the conditioned stimulus.

23   Classical conditioning occurs most effectively when alternative responses are available for the organism.

24   Classical conditioning occurs most effectively when the conditioned responses are strengthened by shaping.

25   Classical conditioning occurs most effectively when the time interval between the conditioned stimulus and unconditioned stimulus is fixed at approximately 0.5 seconds.

26   Gestalt psychology states that the properties of some details in a pattern influence how the whole pattern is perceived.

27   Gestalt psychology states that the properties of the whole pattern affect the way the parts are perceived.

28   Gestalt psychology states that the whole is different from the sum total of its parts.

29   Gestalt psychology deals with the essential characteristics of an actual experience.

30   Gestalt psychology emphasizes the current experiences of the patient in the here and now.

31   The law of closure is a principle of the Gestalt school of perception.

32   The law of continuity is a principle of the Gestalt school of perception.

33   The law of infinity is a principle of the Gestalt school of perception.

34   The law of proximity is a principle of the Gestalt school of perception.

35   The law of similarity is a principle of the Gestalt school of perception.

36   Concerning reinforcement in operant conditioning, variable ratio reinforcement is the easiest to extinguish.

37   Concerning reinforcement in operant conditioning, intermittent reinforcement takes the longest to establish.

38   Fixed ratio reinforcement involves reinforcing after a fixed interval of time of continuous response.

39   Secondary reinforcement involves natural reinforcement through decrease of basic drive.

40   Negative reinforcement can mean reinforcement through withdrawal of aversive conditions.

[Answers on page 85]

Neuropsychology

41   Prosopagnosia is a characteristic feature of dominant occipital lobe lesions.

42   Metamorphopsia is a characteristic feature of dominant occipital lobe lesions.

43   Complex visual hallucination is a clinical feature of dominant occipital lobe lesions.

44   Visuospatial agnosia is a clinical feature of dominant occipital lobe lesions.

45   Finger agnosia is a clinical feature of dominant occipital lobe lesions.

[Answers on page 86]

Human development

46   Basic trust versus mistrust is an essential feature of Piaget's theory of cognitive development.

47   Concrete operational stage is an essential feature of Piaget's theory of cognitive development.

48   Autonomy versus shame and doubt is an essential feature of Piaget's theory of cognitive development.

49   Formal operational stage is an essential feature of Piaget's theory of cognitive development.

50   Sensory motor stage is an essential feature of Piaget's theory of cognitive development.

51   According to attachment theory, babies under the age of 6 months do not manifest attachment behaviours.

52   According to attachment theory, attachment does not occur with people other than the parents.

53   According to attachment theory, feeding is the key factor in establishing attachment.

54   According to attachment theory, attachment is formed equally with mother and father.

55   According to attachment theory, attachment can occur to inanimate objects.

56   Maternal deprivation during early childhood frequently results in developmental delay of language.

57   Maternal deprivation during early childhood frequently results in short stature.

58   Maternal deprivation during infancy frequently results in infantile autism.

59   Maternal deprivation during early childhood results in social disinhibition.

60   Maternal deprivation during early childhood frequently results in shallow relationships with other people.

61   Persistent irregularity in the biological functions is a recognized feature of difficult and temperamental children.

62   Quick and easy adaptation to change is a recognized feature of difficult and temperamental children.

63   A predominantly negative mood is a recognized feature of difficult and temperamental children.

64   There is a threefold risk factor for a behaviour disorder in adulthood in difficult and temperamental children.

65   It is known that difficult and temperamental children show shallow and emotional reactions.

[Answers on page 86]

Assessment, description and measurement of behaviour

66   Psychometric assessment of personality can be made by using the Hostility and the Direction of the Hostility questionnaire (HDHQ).

67   Psychometric assessment of personality can be made by using the General Health Questionnaire (GHQ).

68   Psychometric assessment of personality can be made by using the Symptoms Sign Inventory (SSI).

69   Psychometric assessment of personality can be made by using the California Psychological Inventory (CPI).

70   Psychometric assessment of personality can be made by use of the Rorschach Inkblot Test.

[Answers on page 87]

Basis of psychological treatments

71   According to the psychoanalytic theory of psychosexual development, fixation in the anal phase is related to parsimony in adult life.

72   According to the psychoanalytic theory of psychosexual development, fixation in the anal phase is related to orderliness in adult life.

73   According to the psychoanalytic theory of psychosexual development, fixation in the anal phase is related to obstinacy in adult life.

74   According to the psychoanalytic theory of psychosexual development, fixation in the anal phase is related to frugality in adult life.

75   According to the psychoanalytic theory of psychosexual development, fixation in the anal phase is related to wilfulness in adult life.

76   According to Freud's theory of psychoanalysis, the superego represents the conscience.

77   According to Freud's theory of psychoanalysis, the superego includes unconscious elements.

78   According to Freud's theory of psychoanalysis, the superego may be in conflict with the present values.

79   According to Freud's theory of psychoanalysis, the superego is an accurate replica of a parental figure in early childhood.

80   According to Freud's theory of psychoanalysis, the superego sometimes overlaps with the ego.

81   Anticipation is a mature ego defence mechanism.

82   Altruism is a mature ego defence mechanism.

83   Displacement is a mature ego defence mechanism.

84   Sublimation is a mature ego defence mechanism.

85   Suppression is a mature ego defence mechanism.

86   Ambivalence plays an essential part in the production of hysterical conversion symptoms.

87 Introjection plays an essential part in the production of hysterical conversion symptoms.

88 Reaction formation plays an essential part in the production of hysterical conversion symptoms.

89 Displacement plays an essential part in the production of hysterical conversion symptoms.

90 Denial plays an essential part in the production of hysterical conversion symptoms.

[Answers on page 87]

Social sciences and ethology

91 The sick role, as described by Parsons, stipulates that the sick person has a right to be defined as not responsible for his or her own condition.

92 The sick role, as described by Parsons, stipulates that a sick person has the right to take advantage of any secondary gains involved with being sick.

93 The sick role, as described by Parsons, stipulates that the sick person has the right but not the obligation to define the state of being sick as desirable.

94 The sick role, as described by Parsons, stipulates that the sick person has the right to be exempt from normal social activities.

95 The sick role, as described by Parsons, stipulates that the sick person has the option of seeking competent medical help.

96 High social status is an important model from which observational learning takes place.

97 High social class is an important model from which observational learning takes place.

98 High social power is an important model from which observational learning takes place.

99 High competence is an important model from which observational learning takes place.

100 High integrity is an important model from which observational learning takes place.

101 Improving the image of ethnic minorities in the media is the most effective method of reducing racial prejudice in society.

102 Psychotherapy for black/white confrontations is the most effective method of reducing racial prejudice in society.

103   Interracial contact is the most effective method of reducing racial prejudice in society.

104   Introducing studies of ethnic groups into the school curriculum is an effective method of reducing racial prejudice in society.

105   Legislating against discriminatory behaviour is the most effective method of reducing racial prejudice in society.

106   Ethology is the study of living organisms in their own natural environment.

107   Ethology is useful in understanding human non-verbal behaviour.

108   Ethology can help in understanding the extrapyramidal speech disorders in human beings.

109   Ethology requires a control group for assessment of its effects.

110   Ethology is useful in understanding the process of attachment and separation anxiety.

[Answers on page 88]

Neurosciences

Neuroanatomy

111   The primary motor cortex is in the postcentral gyrus of the parietal lobe.

112   The primary sensory cortex is in the precentral gyrus of the frontal lobe.

113   The visual cortex is in the calcarine fissure of the occipital lobe.

114   The auditory cortex is in the uncus and the parahippocampal gyrus of the temporal lobe.

115   The olfactory cortex is deep within the sylvian fissure in the temporal lobe.

116   As regards neuroglia, the astrocytes are multipolar cells with several thick processes.

117   As regards neuroglia, the glial processes are astrocytes completely covering the outer surfaces of capillaries.

118   Oligodendroglia are small spherical cells with only a few processes.

119   Astrocytes lie in long parallel rows alongside axons.

120   Oligodendroglia form the myelin sheath.

121   Insula is a component of the basal ganglia.

122   Globus pallidus is a component of the basal ganglia.

123   Diencephalon is a component of the basal ganglia.

124   Amygdaloid nucleus is a component of the basal ganglia.

125   Claustrum is a component of the basal ganglia.

126   The pyramidal pathway passes through the tegmentum in the mesencephalon.

127   The pyramidal pathway decussates completely at the medulla oblongata.

128   The pyramidal pathway characteristically degenerates in tabes dorsalis.

129   The pyramidal pathway sends efferents to the ventrolateral nucleus of the thalamus.

130   The pyramidal pathway terminates in the Renshaw cells in the ventral horn of the spinal cord.

131   Broca's motor speech area is a part of the neocortex.

132   The hippocampus is a part of the neocortex.

133   The primary olfactory area is a part of the neocortex.

134   The superior temporal gyrus is a part of the neocortex.

135   The cingulate gyrus is a part of the neocortex.

136   The lower motor neurones lie in the anterior grey column of the spinal cord.

137   The lower motor neurones innervate the muscles of the hand.

138   The lower motor neurones are selectively destroyed in poliomyelitis.

139   The lower motor neurones lie in the posterior grey column of the spinal cord.

140   Lower motor neurones are attacked during an infection by varicella zoster.

141   Neurofibrillary tangles are intracellular structures in the human brain.

142   Senile plaques are intracellular structures in the human brain.

143   Mitochondria are intracellular structures in the human brain.

144   Ependyma is an intracellular structure in the human brain.

145   Nucleolus is an intracellular structure in the human brain.

146   The suprachiasmatic nucleus is a hypothalamic structure.

147   The premammillary nucleus is a hypothalamic structure.

148   The red nucleus is a hypothalamic structure.

149   The paraventricular nucleus is a hypothalamic structure.

150   The olivary nucleus is a hypothalamic structure.

151   The arachnoid membrane is a component of the blood–brain barrier.

152   The endothelial lining of the brain capillaries is a component of the blood–brain barrier.

153   Myelin sheath is a component of the blood–brain barrier.

154   The gliovascular membrane is a component of the blood–brain barrier.

155   Capillary basement is a component of the blood–brain barrier.

156   Blood supply to the internal capsule is provided by the anterior cerebral artery.

157   Blood supply to the internal capsule is provided by the middle cerebral artery.

158   Blood supply to the internal capsule is provided by the posterior cerebral artery.

159   The anterior choroidal artery provides blood to the internal capsule.

160   The internal carotid artery provides blood to the internal capsule.

161   The oculomotor nerve is involved in the generation of the corneal reflex.

162   The optic radiation is involved in the generation of the corneal reflex.

163   The trigeminal nerve is involved in the generation of the corneal reflex.

164   The facial nerve is involved in the generation of the corneal reflex.

165   The spinal nucleus of the trigeminal nerve is involved in the generation of the corneal reflex.

166   The retina is involved in the pupillary reaction.

167   The median forebrain bundle is involved in the pupillary reaction.

168   The optic tracts are involved in the pupillary reaction.

169   The ciliary ganglion is involved in the pupillary reaction.

170   The pupillary sphincter is involved in the pupillary reaction.

[Answers on page 88]

Neuropathology

171   Primary demyelination occurs in Alzheimer's disease.

172   Primary demyelination occurs in Wilson's disease.

173   Primary demyelination occurs in Schilder's disease.

174   Primary demyelination occurs in Tay–Sachs disease.

175   Primary demyelination occurs in multiple sclerosis.

176   Neuropathological studies have shown that the brains of patients with schizophrenia are smaller and lighter compared with normal controls.

177   Neuropathological studies of patients with schizophrenia have shown that the frontal horns of the lateral ventricles are larger than in normal controls.

178   Neuropathological studies of patients with schizophrenia have shown that most abnormalities are present in the basal ganglia, hippocampus and parahippocampal gyrus.

179   Neuropathological studies of patients with schizophrenia have shown that abnormalities are often prominent on the right side of the brain.

180   Neuropathological studies of patients with schizophrenia have shown that changes seen are accompanied by gliosis.

181   Characteristic changes in the brain structure in Alzheimer's disease include localized atrophy of the frontal cortex.

182   Characteristic changes in the brain structure in Alzheimer's disease include widening of sulci.

183   Characteristic changes in the brain structure in Alzheimer's disease include loss of neurones in the basal nucleus of Meynert.

184   Characteristic changes in the brain structure in Alzheimer's disease include loss of dopaminergic neurones from the basal ganglia.

185   Characteristic changes in the brain structure in Alzheimer's disease include innumerable amyloid plaques and neurofibrillary tangles.

186   Neurofibrillary tangles are characteristically seen in Down's syndrome.

187   Neurofibrillary tangles are characteristically seen in Huntington's disease.

188   Neurofibrillary tangles are characteristically seen in Pick's disease.

189   Neurofibrillary tangles are characteristically seen in punch-drunk syndrome.

190   Neurofibrillary tangles are characteristically seen in multi-infarct dementia.

[Answers on page 91]

Neurophysiology

191   An abnormal brain respiratory rate is found in multi-infarct dementia.

192   An abnormal brain respiratory rate is found in delirium tremens.

193   An abnormal brain respiratory rate is found in Wernicke's encephalopathy.

194   An abnormal brain respiratory rate is found in social phobia.

195   An abnormal brain respiratory rate is found in schizophrenia.

196   Features of the action potential of a nerve fibre include reversal of voltage across the nerve membrane.

197   Features of the action potential of a nerve fibre include an inward movement of potassium ions.

198   Features of the action potential of a nerve fibre include an outward movement of chloride ions.

199   Features of the action potential of a nerve fibre include an inward movement of sodium ions.

200   Features of the action potential of a nerve fibre include an outward movement of phosphate ions.

201   G proteins are guanine nucleotide binding proteins.

202   G proteins are embedded in the cellular membrane.

203   G proteins form an intermediate link between receptor and effector enzymes.

204   G proteins are not involved in the adenylate cyclase pathway.

205   G proteins are involved as intermediates in the receptor activated ion channels and other postreceptor pathways.

206   Stimulating the hypothalamus may produce defence reaction arousal in laboratory animals.

207   Stimulating the ventrolateral thalamic nucleus may produce defence reaction arousal in laboratory animals.

208   Stimulating the fornix may produce defence reaction arousal in laboratory animals.

209   Stimulating the hippocampus may produce defence reaction arousal in laboratory animals.

210   Stimulating the globus pallidus may produce defence reaction arousal in laboratory animals.

211   The blood–brain barrier typically separates blood from cerebrospinal fluid and brain.

212   The blood–brain barrier prevents the entry of lipid-soluble substances into the brain cells.

213   The permeability of the blood–brain barrier to drugs is linked to their water solubility.

214   The pH of cerebrospinal fluid can be regulated independently of plasma pH.

215   Large amino acids cross the blood–brain barrier freely.

216   The electroencephalogram of patients with multi-infarct dementia shows little or no activity.

217   The electroencephalogram of patients with delirium tremens shows little or no activity.

218   The electroencephalogram of patients with Alzheimer's disease shows little or no activity.

219   The electroencephalogram of patients with brain death shows little or no activity.

220   The electroencephalogram in patients with Huntington's disease shows little or no activity.

221   The electroencephalogram of a sleeping individual shows sleep spindles at the onset of sleep.

222   The electroencephalogram of a sleeping individual can reveal epileptiform discharges, which are absent in the waking electroencephalogram.

223   The electroencephalogram of a sleeping individual with grand mal epilepsy typically shows direct entry into REM sleep at the onset of sleep.

224   The electroencephalogram of a sleeping individual shows that the total sleep time decreases with advancing age.

225   The electroencephalogram of a sleeping individual reveals marked slow activity with K-complexes in stage 3 of sleep.

226   Short-term anterograde amnesia is more severe with bilateral than unilateral electroconvulsive therapy.

227   Physiological changes associated with the excitement phase of sexual response in women include erection of nipples.

228   Physiological changes associated with the excitement phase of sexual response in women include an increase in sensitivity and withdrawal of the clitoris.

229   Physiological changes associated with the excitement phase of sexual response in women include an increase in the size of the breasts.

230 Physiological changes associated with the excitement phase of sexual response in women include engorgement and spreading of the labia minora and majora.

231 Physiological changes associated with the excitement phase of sexual response in women include an increase in skin temperature.

232 Penile tumescence (as measured by plethysmometry) is considered to be the most reliable measure of arousal state.

233 Up to 50 per cent of patients with cyclothymia will ultimately develop bipolar affective disorder.

234 Evidence that monoamines are involved in the pathogenesis of mood disorders includes the fact that reserpine induces depression in some patients.

235 Evidence that monoamines are involved in the pathogenesis of mood disorders includes the fact sodium valproate is an effective treatment of mania.

236 Evidence that monoamines are involved in the pathogenesis of mood disorders includes the fact that fluoxetine is an effective treatment of depression.

237 Evidence that monoamines are involved in the pathogenesis of mood disorders includes the fact that iproniazid improves mood in patients with tuberculosis.

238 The dexamethasone suppression test is a sensitive screening tool for major depressive disorder.

239 The dexamethasone suppression test is a selective screening tool for major depressive disorder.

240 The dexamethasone suppression test (DST) explains why hypothyroidism is associated with depressive symptoms.

241 The dexamethasone suppression test differentiates non-psychotic depressed patients from those with psychosis.

[Answers on page 92]

Neuroendocrinology

242 Growth hormone inhibits peripheral production of the insulin-like growth factor (IGF-1).

243 Somatostatin has an indirect inhibitory influence on the production of growth hormone.

244 Somatostatin exerts a tonic inhibitory influence on growth hormone.

245　Hypothyroidism leads to severe suppression of growth hormone production in the pituitary gland.

246　Corticosteroids increase the production and release of growth hormone.

[Answers on page 93]

Neurochemistry

247　Gamma-aminobutyric acid (GABA) is the main cortical inhibitory neurotransmitter in the brain.

248　The $GABA_B$ receptor has a chloride channel that mediates GABAergic transmission.

249　Antiepileptic drugs act on $GABA_A$ receptors.

250　GABA receptors are widely distributed with high concentrations in the spinal cord.

251　The functions of GABA receptors depend on the presence of GABA transaminase.

252　Rapid eye movement (REM) sleep latency increase is predictive of the antidepressant effect of a drug.

253　Reserpine antagonism is predictive of the antidepressant effect of a drug.

254　Noradrenaline antagonism is predictive of the antidepressant effect of a drug.

255　Enhancement of chloride channel transmission is predictive of the antidepressant effect of a drug.

256　Selective serotonin reuptake inhibition is predictive of the antidepressant effect of a drug.

257　In calcium channels in the neurones, the neurotransmitter release usually depends on calcium.

258　Calcium channels in the neurones close in response to membrane depolarization.

259　According to current scientific knowledge, only one type of calcium channel is known to occur in the neurones.

260　Some of the side effects of antipsychotic drugs can be explained by calcium channel blockade.

261　Calcium channel blockers like nifedipine and verapamil influence neurotransmitter release.

262　With regard to *in vivo* receptor imaging, both magnetic resonance imaging and positron emission tomography are useful techniques

263 With regard to *in vivo* receptor imaging, affinity of psychotropic drugs to receptors can be accurately calculated.

264 With regard to *in vivo* receptor imaging, it has been shown that clozapine has a much higher affinity for D_2 receptors than haloperidol.

265 With regard to *in vivo* receptor imaging, it can be used to provide information on regional localization of receptors.

266 With regard to *in vivo* receptor imaging, flumazenil is used as a high affinity ligand for opiate receptors.

267 Neuroreceptors have recognition sites that occur on the neuronal cell bodies.

268 Neuroreceptors have a lifespan of up to 6 months.

269 Neuroreceptors are synthesized in the synapses of the neurones.

270 Neuroreceptors can be labelled in postmortem brain tissue.

271 Certain psychotropic drugs alter the synthesis of neuroreceptors.

272 The neuronal membrane resists the passage of ions during its resting state.

273 The neuronal membrane maintains the potential difference across its membrane through ion pumps.

274 The neuronal membrane has ion channels for three major ions: Na^+, K^+ and Cl^-.

275 The neuronal membrane has separate channels for ions that move in and those that move out.

276 The neuronal membrane depolarizes with increased negativity of the transmembrane potential.

277 The ion channels in the neuronal membrane are responsible for the action potential.

278 The ion channels in the neuronal membrane are selective for the type of ion to which they are permeable.

279 The ion channels in the neuronal membrane are only chemically activated.

280 The ion channels are only electrically activated.

281 The ion channels open when depolarization reaches the spike threshold.

[Answers on page 93]

Psychopharmacology

Pharmacokinetics

282   With regard to the effects of drugs on human behaviour, stabilometer devices measure sensory function.

283   With regard to the effects of drugs on human behaviour, the Gibson spiral maze test measures central nervous system arousal.

284   With regard to the effects on human behaviour, the Card Sorting Test measures motor function.

285   The placebo effect includes overcoming negative attitudes to drug treatment.

286   The placebo effect entails increasing expectations of drug treatment.

287   The placebo effect entails patients thinking that they are being deprived of something they believe will benefit them.

288   The placebo effect includes amplification of adverse response to treatment withdrawal.

289   Tricyclic antidepressant drugs are poorly bound to plasma proteins.

290   Smoking may inhibit metabolism of tricyclic antidepressant drugs via 2-hydroxylation.

291   Tricyclic antidepressant drugs potentiate the pressor effect of directly acting sympathomimetic amines.

292   Tricyclic antidepressant drugs enhance the antihypertensive effects of adrenergic neurone blocking agents.

293   According to current scientific knowledge, the selective serotonin reuptake inhibitors are rapidly absorbed in the gut.

294   According to current scientific knowledge, serotonin selective reuptake inhibitors reduce both obsessional thinking and compulsive rituals independent of their antidepressant effect.

295   According to current scientific knowledge, serotonin selective reuptake inhibitors reduce both the frequency and intensity of binges in patients with bulimia nervosa.

296   According to current scientific knowledge, selective serotonin reuptake inhibitors may reduce craving in patients with alcohol dependence syndrome.

297   According to current scientific knowledge, serotonin selective reuptake inhibitors reduce the plasma levels of drugs metabolized by oxidative microsomal enzymes in the liver.

298   Lithium passes freely through the glomerular membrane independent of its serum concentration.

299   Renal clearance of lithium is enhanced by sodium depletion.

300   Lithium blocks the development of the supersensitivity which develops in dopamine receptors after long-term administration of antipsychotic drugs.

301   According to current scientific knowledge, the mechanism of action of lithium includes a decrease in sodium/potassium adenosine triphosphatase.

302   A positive family history of bipolar affective disorder is a predictor of a good response to lithium.

[Answers on page 94]

Pharmacodynamics

303   According to current scientific knowledge, risperidone has combined D_1 and 5-hydroxytryptamine 1 (5-HT$_1$) antagonistic properties.

304   Sulpiride has a high affinity for the tuberoinfundibular tract.

305   According to current scientific knowledge, there is a marked increase in the number of opioid receptors following long-term administration of opiates.

306   According to current scientific knowledge, there is a decrease in the functional activity of opioid receptors following long-term administration of opiates.

307   According to current scientific knowledge, physical dependence on opioids leads to an increase in adenylate cyclase activity.

308   According to current scientific knowledge, there is excessive parasympathetic activity associated with abrupt withdrawal in opioid dependent patients.

309   According to current scientific knowledge of physical dependence on opioids, they act on mu and delta receptors.

[Answers on page 95]

Adverse drug reactions

310   Lithium carbonate leads to clinical goitre in the majority of patients taking the drug.

311   In patients taking lithium carbonate, hyperthyroidism is commonly reported.

312   Lithium-induced thyroid dysfunction is usually irreversible.

313 Lithium carbonate has to be discontinued if thyroxine is prescribed concomitantly in hypothyroid patients.

314 If thyroid dysfunction does not occur in the first 6 months of lithium therapy, monitoring of thyroid functions can be discontinued.

315 Lithium-induced neurotoxicity is usually irreversible.

316 Lithium-induced neurotoxicity rarely manifests as pseudotumour cerebri.

317 Lithium-induced neurotoxicity may lead to permanent deficits, more often in females than in males.

318 Lithium-induced neurotoxicity is clinically indistinguishable from an acute overdose of lithium carbonate.

319 Lithium-induced neurotoxicity does not correlate with electroencephalographic changes.

[Answers on page 95]

Drug dependence

320 With regard to benzodiazepine dependence, there is considerable evidence for genetic predisposition in some patients.

321 The clinical picture of benzodiazepine dependence is characteristically different from heroin addiction.

322 With regard to benzodiazepine dependence, the mechanism for persistent withdrawal symptoms is well understood.

323 Ventricular enlargement is a consistent finding on computed tomography (CT) scans in long-term benzodiazepine users.

324 Benzodiazepine dependence is associated with a specific personality profile.

[Answers on page 96]

Genetics

325 Fragile X syndrome occurs only in boys.

326 Lesch–Nyhan syndrome occurs only in boys.

327 Hunter syndrome occurs only in boys.

328 Hyperuricaemia occurs only in boys.

329 Klinefelter's syndrome occurs only in boys.

330 According to current scientific knowledge, Down's syndrome is transmitted by a single recessive gene.

331   According to current scientific knowledge, Klinefelter's syndrome is transmitted by a single recessive gene.

332   According to current scientific knowledge, hyperprolinaemia types I and II are transmitted by a single recessive gene.

333   According to current scientific knowledge, Gaucher's disease is transmitted by a single recessive gene.

334   According to current scientific knowledge, amaurotic idiocy is transmitted by a single recessive gene.

335   According to current scientific knowledge, it is possible to make a prenatal diagnosis of Huntington's disease.

336   According to current scientific knowledge, it is possible to make a prenatal diagnosis of phenylketonuria.

337   According to current scientific knowledge, it is possible to make a prenatal diagnosis of Hartnup's disorder.

338   According to current scientific knowledge, it is possible to make a prenatal diagnosis of Niemann–Pick Disease, groups A and B.

339   According to current scientific knowledge, it is possible to make a prenatal diagnosis of galactosaemia.

340   In Down's syndrome, there is characteristically an extra chromosome 21.

341   There is an increased risk of Alzheimer's disease in patients with Down's syndrome, compared with the general population.

342   The majority of cases of Down's syndrome are due to translocation involving chromosome 21.

343   In Down's syndrome, mental retardation is reversible if an early diagnosis is made.

344   The life expectancy of a person with Down's syndrome is comparable with that of the general population.

345   Congenital cardiac disease is a characteristic feature of Down's syndrome.

346   Brushfield spots are characteristic features of Down's syndrome.

347   A single transverse palmar crease is a characteristic feature of Down's syndrome.

348   Bradycephaly is a characteristic feature of Down's syndrome.

349   Umbilical hernias are a characteristic feature of Down's syndrome.

[Answers on page 96]

Epidemiology

350　In epidemiological research, Feigner's criteria may be used to determine the case level of phenomenology.

351　In epidemiological research, the General Health Questionnaire may be used to determine the case level of phenomenology.

352　In epidemiological research, the Present State Examination may be used to determine the case level of phenomenology.

353　In epidemiological research, the Schedule for Affective Disorders may be used to determine the case level of phenomenology.

354　In epidemiological research, the Research Diagnostic Criteria may be used to determine the case level of phenomenology.

[Answers on page 96]

Statistics and research methodology

355　There are significantly more severely mentally impaired persons than can be accounted for by chance expectancy at the left-hand side of the intelligence scales due to poor socioeconomic status.

356　There are significantly more severely mentally impaired persons than can be accounted for by chance expectancy at the left-hand side of the intelligence scales due to marital discord.

357　There are significantly more severely mentally impaired persons than can be accounted for by chance expectancy at the left-hand side of the intelligence scales due to mutation.

358　There are significantly more severely mentally impaired persons than can be accounted for by chance expectancy at the left hand side of the intelligence scales due to the fact that mentally impaired people have larger families.

359　There are significantly more severely mentally impaired persons than can be accounted for by chance expectancy at the left-hand side of the intelligence scales due to perinatal brain injuries.

360　Sampling procedures designed for standardization of IQ tests involve socioeconomic status.

361　Sampling procedures designed for standardization of IQ tests involve educational achievements.

362　Sampling procedures designed for standardization of IQ tests involve IQ of the parents.

363　Sampling procedures designed for standardization of IQ tests involve chronological age.

364   Sampling procedures designed for standardization of IQ tests involve occupation.

365   The normal distribution of a variable is important in estimating the standard error of mean.

366   The normal distribution of a variable is important in estimating a variance.

367   The normal distribution of a variable is important in estimating percentile indices.

368   The normal distribution of a variable is important in estimating a correlation coefficient.

369   The normal distribution of a variable is important in estimating confidence intervals.

370   Factor analysis is a statistical technique that enables the reduction of interrelationships within a large sample to a small number of independent factors.

371   Factor analysis is a statistical technique that was initially formulated by statisticians.

372   Factor analysis is a statistical technique that has been used successfully to classify mental disorders.

373   Factor analysis assumes that the relation between the variables and the factors is linear.

374   Factor analysis assumes that the variables are liable to random errors.

375   Factor analysis can be used to test the hypothesis that two samples are drawn from the same population.

376   A chi-squared test for independence can be used to test the hypothesis that two samples are drawn from the same population.

377   Principal component analysis can be used to test the hypothesis that two samples are drawn from the same population.

378   Analysis of variance can be used to test the hypothesis that two samples are drawn from the same population.

379   The Mann–Whitney U test can be used to test the hypothesis that two samples are drawn from the same population.

380   In clinical research, samples may be selected by using stratification.

381   In clinical research, samples may be selected by using multiphasic technique.

382   In clinical research, samples may be selected by using double-blind technique.

383 In clinical research, samples may be selected by using multistage technique.

384 In clinical research, samples may be selected by using minimization technique.

385 The placebo reaction in clinical drug trials refers to the patient's tendency to react to the colour, shape and size of the drug preparation.

386 The placebo reaction in clinical drug trials refers to the patient's tendency to describe side effects on the basis of expectancy and mental attitudes even to dummy preparations.

387 The placebo reactions in clinical drug trials can be influenced by a questionnaire of side effects.

388 The placebo reaction in clinical drug trials refers to the tendency to improve in the first 2 weeks of treatment.

389 The placebo reactions in clinical drug trials depend on the seniority of the prescriber.

390 Measuring outcomes in a research study is valuable because it enables comparisons of the effectiveness of different treatments.

391 Measuring outcomes in a research study is valuable because it allows clinical decisions to be made according to scores on short scales.

392 Measuring outcomes in a research study is valuable because it is simpler and more convenient to measure than the method.

393 Measuring outcomes in a research study is valuable because it enables one to improve the effectiveness of new treatments.

394 Measuring outcomes in a research study is valuable because it may help identify carer stress.

[Answers on page 97]

Medical ethics and principles of law

395 With reference to teleology, the central concept is human rights.

396 The therapeutic relationship between the doctor and patient is based on a contractarian model rather than paternalism.

397 In modern times, a contractarian model of doctor–patient relationship in which there is symmetry of power, largely replaces paternalism.

398 In modern times, paternalism is largely replaced by a contractarian model of doctor-patient relationship in which there is symmetry of knowledge.

399 Any undisclosed division of professional fees is unethical in the UK.

400   The Hippocratic Oath guides today's psychiatrists in all possible
        eventualities.

[Answers on page 98]

Answers

Psychology

Basic, behavioural and social psychology

1   True
2   True   Cognitive–behavioural therapy aims at a primary change in cognition followed by a secondary change in behaviour.
3   True
4   True
5   True
6   False
7   True
8   True   Punishment is an aversive stimulus that is presented specifically to reduce the probability of future response.
9   False   Negative reinforcement is the removal of an unpleasant condition, which increases the probability of occurrence of operant behaviour. It increases the likelihood of the response.
10   True
11   False   The relation between the presentation of the conditioned and unconditioned stimuli is important, varying from optimal learning from a fraction of a second to several seconds. Classical conditioning is most often applied to responses mediated by the autonomic nervous system. The reinforcement schedule is required in operant conditioning.
12   True
13   True
14   False
15   False
16   False
17   True
18   False
19   False
20   True
21   True
22   True
23   False
24   False   Shaping is a type of operant conditioning.
25   False
26   False
27   False
28   True
29   True

30   **True**   Gestalt theory was developed in Germany under the influence of seven men, including Max Wertheimer and Kurt Lewin. In terms of motivation, patients learn to recognize their needs at any given time and how those needs might influence their current behaviour.

31   **True**   The whole is greater than the sum of its parts. Other principles include ground differentiation.

32   **True**

33   **False**

34   **True**

35   **True**

36   **False**   Variable ratio is the hardest to extinguish, which is why gambling is difficult to treat.

37   **True**   Fixed ratio reinforcement schedule involves reinforcing, e.g. 1 in 3 correct responses, and involves reinforcing after a fixed interval of time of continuous responses.

38   **False**   A fixed ratio is one in which there is a constant ratio between the number of behaviours and the number of occurrences of the reward.

39   **False**

40   **True**

Neuropsychology

41   **False**   It is the ability to recognize known faces.

42   **False**   It means distortion of objects.

43   **False**

44   **False**

45   **False**   It is seen in Gerstmann's syndrome and dominant parietal lobe lesions.

Human development

46   **False**   It is the first stage of psychosocial development of a child as proposed by Erik Erikson.

47   **True**   It is the stage occurring between the ages of 7 and 12 years.

48   **False**   This is a stage in the psychosocial development of the child occurring between the ages of 1 and 3 years.

49   **True**   This is the last stage, which occurs from the age of 12 years.

50   **True**   This is the first stage in the child's cognitive development.

51   **True**

52   **False**   Attachment is the baby's special relationship with its primary caregivers. It starts developing during the first months after birth. The infant is capable of multiple attachments.

53   **False**

54   **True**

55   **True**

56   **True**

57   **True**

58   **False**   Children with infantile autism resemble emotionally deprived children, but there are distinguishing features in clinical presentation, e.g. abnormalities in play, stereotypes, ritualistic behaviours, insistence on sameness and resistance to change.

59   **True**

60   **True**

61   **True**

62   **False**

63   **True**

64   **True**

65   **False**   10 per cent of the children in the New York longitudinal study were categorized as having a difficult temperament. They are negative, slow to adapt to changes, show withdrawal reactions to novelty and have intense emotional reactions.

Assessment, description and measurement of behaviour

66   **True**

67   **False**   It allows measurement of 18 traits that are part of normal personality, such as achievement, sociability etc.

68   **False**

69   **True**

70   **True**   This is a projective test, which involves a number of inkblots, none of which has any definite meaning.

Basis of psychological treatments

71   **True**

72   **True**

73   **True**

74   **True**

75   **True**

76   **False**

77   **False**

78   **True**

79   **False**

80   **True**   The superego comes into being with the resolution of the Oedipus complex, which leads to a rapid acceleration of the identification process with the parent of the same sex. The identification is based on the child's struggle to repress the instinctual aims. The effort of renunciation gives the superego its prohibiting character.

81   **True**

82   **True**

83   **False**   It is a neurotic defence mechanism.

84   **True**

85   **True**

86   **False**

87 **False**

88 **False**

89 **False**

90 **False**   According to psychoanalytic theory, conversion is caused by repression of unconscious intrapsychic conflict and the conversion of anxiety into a physical symptom.

Social sciences and ethology

91 **True**

92 **False**

93 **False**

94 **True**

95 **False**   Talcott Parsons' formulation of society's expectations about the sick role involves two rights and two obligations. The obligations are to seek medical help and to define the state of being sick as undesirable.

96 **True**

97 **False**

98 **True**

99 **True**

100 **False**

101 **False**

102 **False**

103 **True**   Interracial contact is the most powerful way of decreasing racial prejudice. The other methods are less effective.

104 **False**

105 **False**

106 **True**

107 **True**

108 **False**

109 **True**

110 **True**   Ethology has contributed to the understanding of human behaviour and also emphasized particular avenues of therapeutic approach in psychiatric care.

Neurosciences

Neuroanatomy

111 **False**   The primary motor cortex is in the precentral gyrus of the frontal lobe.

112 **False**   The primary sensory cortex is in the postcentral gyrus of the parietal lobe.

113 **True**

114 **False**   The auditory cortex lies within the sylvian fissure in the temporal lobe.

115 **False**   The olfactory cortex lies within the uncus and parahippocampal gyrus of the temporal lobe.

116 **True**

117 **True**

118 **True**   Oligodendria lie in long parallel rows alongside axons.

119 **False**

120 **True**

121 **False**   Insula, also known as the Island of Reil, is an area of the central cortex.

122 **True**

123 **False**   Diencephalon surrounds the third ventricle and is not a part of the basal ganglia.

124 **True**

125 **True**

126 **False**   It descends through the corona radiata and the internal capsule and passes through the ventral part of the midbrain and medulla oblongata, and travels down the spinal cord.

127 **False**   The pyramidal tracts are crossed motor (lateral corticospinal) tracts unlike the direct or uncrossed motor (anterior corticospinal) tracts. They decussate in the medulla oblongata and pass inferiorly to the opposite side of the spinal cord.

128 **True**   Degeneration of the pyramidal tracts leads to ataxia with a wide-based and stamping gait, loss of vibration and deep pain sensation and positive Romberg's sign.

129 **False**   This high speed and large diameter system connects the cerebral cortex to the ventral horn of the spinal cord, without intervening synapses.

130 **False**   It terminates mainly on interneurones in the dorsal horns of the spinal cord and a small portion terminates directly on the anterior motor neurones. Renshaw cells are inhibitory interneurones in the anterior horn of the spinal cord.

131 **True**

132 **False**   It is a part of the archicortex.

133 **False**   It is a part of the paleocortex.

134 **True**

135 **True**   From a development point of view, the cerebral cortex consists of three parts: paleocortex, archicortex and neocortex, i.e. the new structures. The neocortex becomes prominent in mammals and achieves its greatest development in primates. In human beings, it constitutes about 90 per cent of the cerebral cortex.

136 **True**

137 **True**   The skeletal muscles are innervated by nerves that originate in the lower motor neurones of the anterior grey column and in the motor nuclei of the cranial nerves.

138 **True**   This leads to flaccid paralysis, hypotonia, decreased deep tendon reflexes and muscle wasting in poliomyelitis.

139 **False**

140 **False** In herpes zoster, the cells of the posterior root ganglia are affected, leading to eruptions of vesicles and change in the colour of skin in the affected area.

141 **True** They are intracellular paired helical filaments seen in the hippocampus, amygdala, neocortex, locus coeruleus, and nucleus of Meynert and raphe nuclei.

142 **False** They are characterized by the deposition of beta-A_4 protein, which is an abnormal fragment of the amyloid precursor protein, in the extracellular space. The gene is on chromosome 21.

143 **True**

144 **False** Ependyma are a type of interstitial brain cells, which make up most of the nervous tissue. Other cells include astrocytes, oligodendrocytes and microglia.

145 **True**

146 **True**

147 **True**

148 **False**

149 **True**

150 **False**

151 **True**

152 **True**

153 **False** It is a lamellated interrupted membrane covering the axon of a nerve cell.

154 **True**

155 **True** The blood–brain barrier is responsible for preventing rapid equilibrium of some drugs between the blood, on one side, and the brain and cerebrospinal fluid on the other. The normal operation of the blood–brain barrier may alter in the presence of acute cerebral lesions, e.g. infection.

156 **True** It supplies the inferior half of the anterior limb.

157 **True** It supplies the superior halves of the anterior and posterior limbs of the internal capsule.

158 **False**

159 **True** It supplies the posterior two-thirds of the posterior limbs of the internal capsule.

160 **True** The posterior communicating branch of the internal carotid artery supplies the anterior one-third of the posterior limb of the internal capsule.

161 **False**

162 **False**

163 **True** It provides the afferent path of the corneal reflex.

164 **True** It provides the efferent path of the corneal reflex.

165 **True** Along with the spinal nucleus of the facial nerve, it provides the central path in neurotransmission.

166 **True**

167 **False** It consists of ascending noradrenergic, dopaminergic and serotonergic fibres terminating in higher brain areas.

168 True
169 True
170 True

Neuropathology

171 False   Global atrophy of the brain is mainly due to neuronal loss, shrinkage of dendritic branching and a reactive astrocytosis in the cerebral cortex.

172 False   The main changes are widespread copper deposition in the central nervous system, particularly marked in the basal ganglia.

173 True

174 False   The condition is caused by the absence of a vital enzyme called hexosaminidase A, which may lead to secondary demyelination.

175 True

176 True

177 False

178 True

179 False

180 False   No characteristic neuropathological abnormality has yet been found in the brains of patients with schizophrenia. There is a growing consensus that temporal horns of the lateral ventricles are enlarged and abnormalities are prominent on the left side of the brain.

181 False   There is generalized atrophy of the cerebral cortex with widening of the sulci and enlargement of the ventricles.

182 True

183 True   It is the most striking feature of Alzheimer's disease.

184 False   Acetylcholine neurones are mainly affected.

185 True

186 True

187 False   Histopathological changes include neuronal loss in the cerebral cortex, particularly affecting the frontal lobes and gamma-aminobutyric acid (GABA) neurones in the corpus callosum.

188 False   A characteristic histological feature is the presence of argyrophilic intracytoplasmic neuronal inclusion bodies, known as Pick's bodies. These consist of paired helical filaments and endoplasmic reticulum, which stain positively with silver stains, antibodies to ubiquitin and most particularly to tau.

189 True   There are multiple cerebral infarcts with local or general atrophy of the brain and secondary ventricular dilatation.

190 False   Other conditions associated with neurofibrillary tangles include postencephalitic parkinsonism, the parkinsonism–dementia complex of Guam, amyotrophic lateral sclerosis, progressive supranuclear palsy and patients who have received aluminium through renal dialysis.

Neurophysiology

191 **True**

192 **True**

193 **True**

194 **False**

195 **False**

196 **True**

197 **False** Movement of potassium ions out of the membrane increases.

198 **False** Chloride ions are not involved in an action potential.

199 **True** An action potential is a self-propagating transmembrane current that occurs when the intraneuronal electrical potential reaches its threshold. The passage of an action potential along a neuronal axon is an all or none phenomenon.

200 **False** Phosphate ions are not involved in action potential.

201 **True** G proteins are so named because they require guanosine triphosphate (GTP) for their action. They are sometimes referred to as the N proteins for nucleotide binding regulatory protein.

202 **True**

203 **True**

204 **False** They affect the activity of adenylate cyclase, which, when active, converts adenosine triphosphate (ATP) into cyclic adenosine monophosphate (AMP).

205 **True**

206 **True** Such a reaction is produced by stimulation of the limbic system.

207 **False** The anterior nucleus of the thalamus is part of the limbic system.

208 **True**

209 **True**

210 **False** The globus pallidus is a part of the basal ganglia.

211 **True**

212 **False** Lipid-soluble substances pass readily through the blood–brain barrier.

213 **False** As above.

214 **True** The pH of cerebrospinal fluid can be regulated independently of plasma pH, because unionized carbon dioxide passes across the blood–brain barrier much more readily than bicarbonate ions.

215 **True**

216 **False**

217 **False** There may be diffuse irregularity and excess fast activity.

218 **False**

219 **True**

220 **False** The amplitude is often, but not invariably, reduced.

221 **False** Alpha spindles are present in stage 1 whereas sleep spindles of fast activity are present in stage 2 of sleep.

222 **True** Grand mal seizures are activated in non-rapid eye movement (REM) sleep, while absences or minor seizures may be seen in REM sleep.

223 False   Seen in narcolepsy.
224 True
225 True
226 True   It affects the ability to learn new information. It resolves rapidly and usually completely by 6 months.
227 True
228 False
229 True
230 True
231 True
232 True
233 True
234 True
235 False
236 True
237 True
238 False
239 False
240 False
241 False

Neuroendocrinology

242 False   It stimulates the production of insulin-like growth factor.
243 False   Somatostatin has a direct inhibitory influence on the production of growth hormone.
244 True
245 True
246 True

Neurochemistry

247 True
248 False $GABA_B$ receptors are linked to calcium or potassium channels.
249 True $GABA_A$ receptors are linked to chloride channels.
250 True
251 True
252 True
253 True
254 True
255 False   Chloride channels are implicated in the mechanism of action of anxiolytic drugs.
256 True
257 True
258 False
259 False
260 True

261 **False**   Calcium channels open in response to membrane depolarization. They are subdivided into a low-voltage activator and a high-voltage activator, which are further divided into two subtypes. The calcium channel blockers do not influence neurotransmitter release.

262 **False**   Only positron emission tomography is useful for *in vivo* receptor imaging.

263 **True**

264 **False**   Clozapine occupancy is only partial (37 per cent), whereas it is 85 per cent with haloperidol.

265 **True**

266 **False**   Labelled flumazenil is used for benzodiazepine receptors.

267 **False**   Receptor recognition sites occur at synapses.

268 **False**   Lifespan of receptors varies from 7 to 30 days.

269 **False**   Receptors are synthesized in the cell bodies of neurones and transported down the axon into the target sites on the cell membrane.

270 **True**

271 **True**

272 **True**

273 **True**

274 **False**   For four major ions, the fourth being Ca^{2+}.

275 **False**

276 **False**   Depolarization occurs with decreased negativity.

277 **True**

278 **False**   They can be activated both electrically and chemically. The electrically activated channels are also called 'voltage sensitive'.

279 **True**

280 **False**

281 **False**   Only those ion channels responsible for the action potential open when the depolarization reaches the spike threshold.

Psychopharmacology

Pharmacokinetics

282 **False**   These assess motor function and balance. Other measures of ballistic activity include finger tapping.

283 **False**   This assesses sensorimotor function. Other tests include pursuit rotor test, card sorting, reaction time and measurement of saccadic eye movements.

284 **False**   This assesses sensorimotor function.

285 **False**   The doctor overcoming negative attitudes to drug treatment helps to produce a placebo effect.

286 **True**

287 **True**

288 **True**

289 **False**   Extensively bound to plasma proteins, e.g. imipramine is 75–95 per cent protein bound.

290 **False**   Smoking and barbiturates facilitate the metabolism of tricyclic antidepressant drugs.

291 **True**

292 **False**   They inhibit the antihypertensives probably by blocking the uptake of these drugs into the sympathetic nerve terminals (e.g. guanethidine).

293 **False**   Slowly but completely absorbed by the gut.

294 **True**

295 **True**

296 **True**

297 **False**

298 **True**

299 **False**

300 **True**

301 **False**

302 **True**

Pharmacodynamics

303 **False**   It is a D_2 and 5-HT_2 antagonist. It also has noradrenergic and histamine blocking actions, but no anticholinergic effects.

304 **True**   It causes galactorrhoea.

305 **False**   No significant change.

306 **True**

307 **False**   A decrease in adenylate activity is indicative of a decrease in the functional activity of opioid receptors.

308 **False**   Excessive sympathetic activity.

309 **True**

Adverse drug reactions

310 **False**   Thyroid goitre occurs in a small percentage of patients.

311 **False**   It is rare, suggesting that the cases may be coincidental.

312 **False**

313 **False**   Thyroxine can be prescribed together with lithium.

314 **False**   All patients on lithium require monitoring of thyroid functions at least annually.

315 **False**   It is usually reversible with withdrawal of the drug.

316 **True**

317 **True**

318 **True**

319 **False**   Correlation is better with electroencephalography, while there is post-correlation with serum levels.

Drug dependence

320 **True**
321 **True**
322 **False**
323 **False**
324 **True**

Genetics

325 **False**   Female carriers of fragile X syndrome may manifest the typical physical characteristics, e.g. large head and ears, long narrow face and short stature.
326 **True**
327 **True**
328 **True**
329 **True**
330 **False**   It is the commonest autosomal abnormality of trisomy 21 due to non-disjunction and translocation.
331 **False**   It is a sex chromosome abnormality in which phenotype males possess more than one X chromosome per somatic cell nucleus.
332 **True**
333 **True**
334 **True**
335 **True**   It is transmitted as an autosomal dominant gene on the G8 fragment of chromosome 4.
336 **False**   It is an autosomal recessive disorder due to a defect of phenylalanine hydroxylase.
337 **False**   It is an autosomal recessive disorder involving the transport of certain amino acids in the intestines and kidneys.
338 **True**   It is a defect of sphingomyelinase.
339 **True**   It is a defect of galactose 1-phosphate uridyl transferase.
340 **True**
341 **True**
342 **False**   The majority of cases are due to trisomy 21, a non-disjunction during meiosis.
343 **False**   It is always irreversible.
344 **False**   It is usually less than that of the general population.
345 **False**   It is an associated feature in some patients.
346 **True**
347 **True**
348 **True**
349 **False**   There is an increased incidence of umbilical hernias.

Epidemiology

350 **True**
351 **True**

352 **True**

353 **True**

354 **True** All these instruments measure different types of phenomenology, e.g. Feighner's criteria are used for the diagnosis of depression.

Statistics and research methodology

355 **True**

356 **False**

357 **False**

358 **False** Large families have more individuals with mental impairments (learning disabilities) than their fair share, but mentally impaired people do not necessarily have large families.

359 **True**

360 **True**

361 **True**

362 **False**

363 **True**

364 **True** The intelligence quotient (IQ) is the ratio of mental age over chronological age, multiplied by 100, doing away with the decimal point. IQ is a measure of present functioning ability and not necessarily of future potential.

365 **True**

366 **True**

367 **True**

368 **True**

369 **True**

370 **True**

371 **False** Psychologists formulated it.

372 **True**

373 **True**

374 **True**

375 **True**

376 **True**

377 **True**

378 **True**

379 **False** The Mann–Whitney U test is essentially a test of significance.

380 **True**

381 **True**

382 **False** Double-blind refers to the design of the study, where both the observer and the patient are unaware of the independent variables when measuring dependent variables.

383 **True**

384 **True**

385 **True**

386 **True**

387 **True**

388 **True**   A significant placebo response may occur within the first 2 weeks in antidepressant drug trials. This is not necessarily true for trials with other drugs.

389 **False**

390 **True**

391 **False**

392 **False**

393 **True**

394 **True**

Medical ethics and principles of law

395 **False**   The central concept is people's interests, whether these are concerns, desires or needs. Fulfilment or frustration of these interests is the ultimate source of value.

396 **True**

397 **True**   Yes, a contractarian model of relationship between the doctor and the patient replaces paternalism.

398 **False**   Asymmetry of knowledge but symmetry of power.

399 **True**   British Medical Association (1981) The Handbook of Medical Ethics. London: British Medical Association; World Medical Association (1948) General Assembly, Geneva (amended 1968, Sydney, and 1983, Venice); World Psychiatric Association (1977) (revised 1983) General Assembly, Hawaii.

400 **False**   The Oath cannot possibly guide present day psychiatrists struggling with concepts that were probably not anticipated by Hippocrates and his peers. The Oath is a blunt list of dos and don'ts without an argued basis, which could be extended to modern practice.

10 BASIC SCIENCES: PAPER 3 (ISQs)

Sample questions

Psychology

Basic, behavioural and social psychology

1   According to extrinsic motivation theory, needs activate drives.

2   According to extrinsic motivation theory, drive reduction has reinforcing properties for learning a new behaviour.

3   According to extrinsic motivation theory, needs originate from biological homoeostasis.

4   According to extrinsic motivation theory, needs arise out of physiological homoeostatic imbalance.

5   According to extrinsic motivation theory, secondary drives are acquired by learning.

6   Eysenck is linked with idiographic theories of personality.

7   Kelly is linked with idiographic theories of personality.

8   Cattell is linked with idiographic theories of personality.

9   Rogers is linked with idiographic theories of personality.

10   Reich is linked with idiographic theories of personality.

[Answers on page 120]

Neuropsychology

11   Benton's Verbal Fluency Test is used to assess frontal lobe functions.

12   The Wisconsin Card Sorting Test is useful in assessing frontal lobe functions.

13   Benton's Visual Retention Test is useful in assessing parietal lobe functions.

14   The Complex Figure of Rey is useful in assessing temporal lobe functions.

15   Wechsler's Adult Intelligence Scale–Revised assesses auditory concentration.

[Answers on page 120]

Human development

16   According to Freud's theory of psychosexual development, fixation in the oral stage is related to narcissism in adult life.

17   According to Freud's theory of psychosexual development, fixation in the oral stage is related to stubbornness in adult life.

18   According to Freud's theory of psychosexual development, fixation in the oral stage is related to excessive optimism in adult life.

19   According to Freud's theory of psychosexual development, fixation in the oral stage is related to pessimism in adult life.

20   According to Freud's theory of psychosexual development, fixation in the oral stage is related to 'identity confusion' in adult life.

21   Separation anxiety is an essential feature of Erik Erikson's theory of psychosocial development.

22   Initiative versus guilt is an essential feature of Erik Erikson's theory of psychosocial development.

23   Industry versus inferiority is an essential feature of Erik Erikson's theory of psychosocial development.

24   The preoperational stage is an essential feature of Erik Erikson's theory of psychosocial development.

25   Identity versus role confusion is an essential feature of Erik Erikson's theory of psychosocial development.

26   Piaget's preoperational stage of cognitive development includes characteristic egocentrism.

27   Piaget's preoperational stage of cognitive development includes mastery of conservation.

28   According to Piaget's preoperational stage of cognitive development rules are inviolate.

29   Piaget's preoperational stage of cognitive development includes ability to detach logic from immediate experience.

30   Piaget's preoperational stage of cognitive development includes animism.

31   The unified theory of Maslow involves both love and belonging.

32   The unified theory of Maslow involves competence.

33   The unified theory of Maslow involves autonomy.

34   The unified theory of Maslow involves curiosity.

35   The unified theory of Maslow involves self-esteem.

36   Puberty usually occurs earlier in boys than in girls.

37   Adolescent turmoil is considered to be essential for healthy adolescent development.

38   Adolescents rarely identify with their parental values.

39   Acquisition of formal operational thoughts occurs during adolescence.

40   School age adolescents tend to be mainly in groups of the same sex.

[Answers on page 120]

Assessment, description and measurement of behaviour

41   Research on medical students' psychiatric interviewing techniques reveals that they enthusiastically elicit the sexual history.

42   Research on medical students' psychiatric interviewing techniques reveals that they frequently interrupt patients.

43   Research on medical students' psychiatric interviewing techniques reveals that they are often afraid to look at the watch or clock in case this upsets the patient.

44   Research on medical students' interviewing techniques reveals that the patients usually accept jargon.

45   Research on medical students' interviewing techniques reveals that non-verbal cues are usually picked up.

46   The Present State Examination provides an operational definition of each symptom to be rated.

47   The Present State Examination provides no criteria for severity of symptoms.

48   The Present State Examination can be used to characterize mental disorders.

49   The American version of Present State Examination is called the Schedule for Affective Disorders and Schizophrenia.

50   The Schedule for Affective Disorders and Schizophrenia is identical to the Present State Examination in the scope of its application in clinical practice.

51   With regard to the features of the measurement instruments of attitude, the Thurstone Scale is a scale where the subject is presented with a number of statements.

52   In the Likert Scale for measurement of attitude, the subject is presented with a range of statements and they tick those with which they agree.

53   The Likert Scale is more sensitive than the Thurstone Scale for measuring attitude.

54   With regard to the measurement instruments of attitude, semantic differential is where a series of two evaluative adjectives or verbs, each at either end of a line act as a visual analogue scale.

55   With regard to the measurement instruments of attitude, Lie scales are used to counter the problem of social desirability set answers.

[Answers on page 121]

Basis of psychological treatments

56   Identification is an example of immature ego defence mechanisms.

57   Inhibition is an example of immature ego defence mechanisms.

58   Intellectualization is an example of immature ego defence mechanisms.

59   Introjection is an example of immature ego defence mechanisms.

60   Isolation is an example of immature ego defence mechanisms.

[Answers on page 122]

Social sciences and ethology

61   Cognitive dissonance arises when there is palpable disparity between two behavioural elements.

62   Resolution of cognitive dissonance leads to decreased internal discomfort.

63   Cognitive dissonance results in self-deception.

64   Cognitive dissonance is usually found in patients with schizophrenia.

65   Cognitive dissonance leads to attitude changes.

66   Ethnic differences in response to pain are attributed mainly to experimental bias.

67   Ethnic differences in response to pain are attributed mainly to intellectual ability to understand the significance of the disease.

68   Ethnic differences in response to pain are attributed mainly to differences in subjective experience of pain.

69   Ethnic differences in response to pain are attributed mainly to cultural stoicism or emotionalism.

70   Ethnic differences in response to pain are attributed mainly to differences in tolerance threshold.

71   Cognitive dissonance deals with people striving for consistency between cognitions which they think are related.

72   Cognitive dissonance can arise out of conflicting expectations.

73   Cognitive dissonance is experienced as uncomfortable and leads to attempts to reduce it.

74   With regard to cognitive dissonance, the less important the cognition, the more powerful the dissonance.

75   Dismissing information creating dissonance in the first place may reduce cognitive dissonance.

76   A characteristic feature of type A personality is extreme competitiveness.

77   A characteristic feature of type A personality is needed for peer approval.

78   A characteristic feature of type A personality is explosiveness of speech.

79   Type A personality is associated with a lower risk of myocardial infarction.

80   A characteristic feature of Type A personality is striving for achievement.

81   The ethological concept of imprinting has made a significant contribution to the understanding of human behaviour.

82   The ethological concept of critical period has made a significant contribution to the understanding of human behaviour.

83   The ethological concept of fixed action pattern has made a significant contribution to the understanding of human behaviour.

84   The ethological concept of ethnic bonds has made a significant contribution to the understanding of human behaviour.

85   The ethological concept of sign stimulus has made a significant contribution to the understanding of human behaviour.

[Answers on page 122]

Neurosciences

Neuroanatomy

86   As regards the functions of neuroglia, astrocytes help to form the blood–brain barrier.

87   As regards the functions of neuroglia, microglia are phagocytic.

88   Astrocytes are involved in phagocytosis.

89   Schwann cells form the myelin sheath of central neurones.

90   Ependyma cells line the central canal of the spinal cord.

91   The middle cerebral artery is a branch of the circle of Willis.

92   The anterior choroidal artery is a branch of the circle of Willis.

93   The ophthalmic artery is a branch of the circle of Willis.

94   The anterior inferior cerebellar artery is a branch of the circle of Willis.

95   The posterior communicating artery is a branch of the circle of Willis.

96   The optic chiasma is situated anterior to the pituitary stalk.

97   The optic chiasma is situated lateral to the internal carotid artery.

98   The optic chiasma is a cross junction of both sensory and motor nerve fibres.

99   The optic chiasma receives axons from the bipolar cells of the retina.

100   The optic chiasma is responsible for bilateral vision in both eyes.

101   Complete or partial occlusion of the posterior cerebral artery leads to alexia without agraphia.

102   Complete or partial occlusion of the anterior cerebral artery leads to contralateral paresis of upper limb only.

103   Complete or partial occlusion of the middle cerebral artery leads to contralateral hemianopsia.

104   Complete or partial occlusion of the basilar artery leads to locked-in syndrome.

105   Complete or partial occlusion of the posterior inferior cerebellar artery leads to Horner's syndrome.

106   In the cerebral cortex, the paleocortex consists of five layers.

107   The neocortex consists of six layers.

108   The neocortex has five basic types of neurone.

109   The limbic system is a part of the paleocortex.

110   The horizontal cells of Cajal form the innermost layer of the neocortex.

111   The auditory pathway sends efferents to the superior temporal gyrus.

112   With regard to the auditory pathway, the sensory receptors are in the organ of Corti.

113   With regard to the auditory pathway, damage to the internal capsule can cause unilateral deafness.

114   With regard to the auditory pathway, unilateral lesions of Heschl's gyrus are accompanied by unilateral deafness.

115   With regard to the auditory pathway, low frequency sounds are relayed in the superior olivary complex.

116   The association areas of the cerebral cortex are divided into primary and secondary areas.

117   With regard to the association areas of the cerebral cortex, the secondary areas have more wide spread projections.

118   The association areas of the cerebral cortex receive input from the relay nuclei of thalamus.

119   The association areas of the cerebral cortex perform an integrative function.

120   The association areas of the cerebral cortex form a much larger proportion of the cortex in comparison to the primary motor and sensory cortices.

121   The optic nerve is involved in the production of the pupillary light reflex.

122   The optic radiation is involved in the production of the pupillary light reflex.

123   The Edinger–Westphal nucleus is involved in the production of the pupillary light reflex.

124   The occipital cortex is involved in the production of the pupillary light reflex.

125   The oculomotor nuclei are involved in the production of the pupillary light reflex.

126   Dendrites do not contain mitochondria.

127   Dendrites are covered by myelin sheath.

128   Dendrites are found only in the brain.

129   Dendrites act as synaptic plates.

130   Dendrites bear spikes that act as sites for synaptic contact.

131   Red nucleus is a part of the mesolimbic tract.

132   Substantia nigra is a part of the mesolimbic tract.

133   Amygdala is a part of the mesolimbic tract.

134   Caudate nucleus is a part of the mesolimbic tract.

135   Fornix is a part of the mesolimbic tract.

[Answers on page 123]

Neuropathology

136   In Alzheimer's disease, the plaques are composed of paired helical filaments.

137   In Alzheimer's disease, the tangles consist of amyloid precursor protein deposits.

138   In Alzheimer's disease, Hirano bodies are eosinophilic cigar-shaped bodies.

139   In Alzheimer's disease, there is cellular loss in the basal magnocellular nucleus of Meynert.

140   In Alzheimer's disease, amyloid deposition occurs in ventricular walls.

141   Wilson's disease is a recognized cause of subcortical dementia.

142   Huntington's disease is a recognized cause of subcortical dementia.

143   Acquired immune deficiency syndrome (AIDS)–dementia complex is a recognized cause of subcortical dementia.

144   Normal pressure hydrocephalus is a recognized cause of subcortical dementia.

145   Parkinson's disease is a recognized cause of subcortical dementia.

146   The neuropathological changes in multiple sclerosis usually show that the plaques develop along the course of small veins.

147   The neuropathological changes in multiple sclerosis show disruption of the blood–brain barrier.

148   The neuropathological changes in multiple sclerosis show that white matter changes as seen on magnetic resonance imaging (MRI) occur only in periventricular areas.

149   The neuropathological changes in multiple sclerosis show astrocytic gliosis.

150   The neuropathological changes in multiple sclerosis show predominant lesions in the white matter of the brain.

151   Neuropathological changes in prion dementia include status spongiosus.

152   Neuropathological changes in Huntington's disease include atrophy of the head of the caudate nucleus and putamen.

153   Neuropathological changes in herpes simplex encephalitis include petechial haemorrhages in the mamillary bodies.

154   Neuropathological changes in Pick's disease include Hirano bodies.

155   Lewy bodies are found in dementia of frontal lobe type.

[Answers on page 124]

Neurophysiology

156   Defence reaction arousal in laboratory animals may be produced by stimulating the cingulate gyrus.

157   Stimulating the stria terminalis may produce a defence reaction arousal in laboratory animals.

158   Defence reaction arousal in laboratory animals may be produced by stimulating the anterior thalamus.

159   Stimulating the dentate gyrus may produce a defence reaction arousal in laboratory animals.

160   Defence reaction arousal in laboratory animals may be produced by stimulating the amygdaloid body.

161   Benzodiazepine drugs produce an increase in fast beta activity on the electroencephalogram.

162   Lithium carbonate is associated with diffuse slow activity on the electroencephalogram.

163   Monoamine oxide inhibitor drugs produce insignificant effects on the electroencephalogram.

164   The tricyclic antidepressant drugs produce an increase in delta and theta activity on the electroencephalogram.

165   Lithium carbonate produces disorganization of background rhythm on the electroencephalogram.

166   Concerning the energy metabolism of the brain, it can use lipids and proteins for energy.

167   The brain has large stores of glycogen.

168   The brain can use ketone bodies for energy under certain circumstances.

169   The energy metabolism of the brain differs from other tissues because of increased activity of the 'gamma-aminobutyric acid shunt' pathway.

170   The cerebral metabolic rate declines in Alzheimer's disease.

171   Rapid eye movement (REM) sleep represents more than 50 per cent of total sleep time in neonates.

172   Most of the human growth hormone is secreted during REM sleep.

173   The body shows decreased metabolic rate during slow-wave sleep.

174   Benzodiazepine drugs suppress slow-wave sleep.

175   Tricyclic antidepressant drugs suppress REM sleep.

176   Proteins readily enter the brain through the blood–brain barrier.

177   Lipid-soluble substances pass slowly into the brain.

178   The blood–brain barrier regulates the movement of substances in and out of the brain.

179   The blood–brain barrier is facilitated by gaps between the cells of the capillary endothelium.

180   The blood–brain barrier is only a functional rather than an actual barrier.

181   The blood–brain barrier bypasses hepatic metabolism.

182   The blood–brain barrier ultimately depends on the permeability of the capillary membrane.

183   With regard to the blood–brain barrier, it mainly occurs at the cerebellar tentorial level.

184   The blood–brain barrier is a selectively permeable system.

185   The blood–brain barrier is guided by the 'pH partition hypothesis'.

186   The electroencephalogram pattern significantly alters during hypnosis.

187   The electroencephalogram pattern usually does not change with maturation after the age of 10 years.

188   The electroencephalogram is characteristically altered during treatment with selective serotonin reuptake inhibitors.

189   The electroencephalogram pattern remains abnormal for at least 3 months following a six-treatment course of electroconvulsive therapy (ECT).

190   The electroencephalographic pattern in a newborn full-term baby is characterized by a relative absence of electrical activity.

191   Alpha rhythm is most prominent over the occipital lobe in the electroencephalogram.

192   With regard to an electroencephalogram, low frequency and high amplitude activities are predominantly noticed in waking adults.

193   Opening the eyes results in attenuation of alpha rhythm on electroencephalography.

194   The electroencephalogram exhibits desynchronization in the superficial layers of the cerebral cortex.

195   Normal electroencephalographic rhythms do not vary after the age of 20 years.

196   Structural imaging in bipolar affective disorder shows enlarged ventricles and amygdala, and prominent sulci.

197   Structural imaging in bipolar affective disorder usually shows smaller medial prefrontal cortex.

198   The dexamethasone suppression test usually shows non-suppression of cortisol in depressed patients.

199   Manic episodes are associated with increased platelet monoamine levels.

200   Manic episodes are associated with increased serum cortisol levels.

201   Manic episodes are associated with a reduction in thyroid stimulating hormone response to thyroid releasing factor.

202   Manic episodes are associated with increased glucose tolerance.

203   Manic episodes are associated with diffuse abnormalities on electroencephalographic recordings.

204   With regard to neurophysiology of sleep, wakefulness in maintained by activity of the ascending reticular activating system.

205   The onset of sleep is due to decrease in reticular activating system activity.

206   Approximately 25 per cent of total sleep time is made up of rapid eye movement (REM).

207   High frequency (12–14 Hz) sleep spindles occur in stage II of sleep.

208   Stage IV and total sleep time decrease in the elderly.

209   Benzodiazepines suppress stage IV of sleep.

210   Suppression of REM sleep occurs in the early part of night, with chronic benzodiazepine use.

211   On withdrawal of benzodiazepines, a rebound increase above the 'normal' amount of REM sleep occurs.

212   It may take up to 6 weeks to see a return to normal sleep pattern on benzodiazepine withdrawal.

213   Barbiturates are more likely to suppress REM sleep than benzodiazepines.

[Answers on page 125]

Neuroendocrinology

214   Increased plasma osmolality acts as a stimulus for release of pituitary hormones.

215   There is a nocturnal surge of growth hormone during fast-wave sleep.

216   Stimulated serum growth hormone levels are usually lower in premenopausal than postmenopausal women.

217 Noradrenaline does not cross the blood–brain barrier.

218 As regards peptides, starvation leads to increased cerebrospinal fluid levels of endorphins in patients with anorexia nervosa.

[Answers on page 126]

Neurochemistry

219 Glutamate and aspartate are excitatory amino acid neurotransmitters.

220 Excitatory amino acid neurotransmitters act on N-methyl-D-aspartate (NMDA) receptors.

221 Excitatory amino acid neurotransmitters act on kainite and quisqualate receptors.

222 Excitatory amino acid neurotransmitters play an important role in learning and memory.

223 Excitatory amino acid neurotransmitters are found to lead to hyperpolarization in neurones.

224 Glutamate is a monoamine neurotransmitter.

225 Dopamine is a monoamine neurotransmitter.

226 Glycine is a monoamine neurotransmitter.

227 Histamine is a monoamine neurotransmitter.

228 Gamma-aminobutyric acid (GABA) is a monoamine neurotransmitter.

229 As regards muscarinic (m) receptors, M_1 receptors are concentrated in the sympathetic ganglia, corpus striatum and stomach.

230 Muscarinic (m) receptors are closely associated with sodium channels.

231 Pilocarpine is an agonist at muscarinic receptors.

232 Decamethonium and succinylcholine are muscarinic receptor antagonists.

233 Muscarinic receptor antagonists have both central and peripheral actions.

234 As regards the dopamine hypothesis of schizophrenia, all known effective antipsychotic compounds block dopamine receptors both *in vivo* and *in vitro*.

235 As regards the dopamine hypothesis of schizophrenia, amphetamines in high doses produce a psychosis resembling paranoid schizophrenia.

236 As regards the dopamine hypothesis of schizophrenia, cerebrospinal fluid of patients with schizophrenia shows significantly decreased levels of metabolites of dopamine.

237 According to the dopamine hypothesis of schizophrenia, oral administration of dopamine in normal subjects produces a psychosis similar to schizophrenia.

238 All drugs effective in the treatment of schizophrenia invariably raise prolactin levels.

239 Anticholinesterases inhibit the enzyme acetyl cholinesterase.

240 L-Dopa is an example of an anticholinesterase.

241 Physostigmine is an example of an anticholinesterase.

242 Anticholinesterases may benefit patients with Alzheimer's disease.

243 Anticholinesterases lead to accumulation of acetylcholine at cholinergic synapses.

244 G-protein coupled receptors are distinct from the effector proteins.

245 G-protein coupled receptors have extracellular recognition sites for ligands.

246 G-protein coupled receptors link cell surface receptors to a variety of enzymes and ion channels.

247 G-protein coupled receptors can increase in number after blocking by antagonistic compounds.

248 G-protein coupled receptors effect action only through the adenyl cyclase second messenger system.

249 With reference to interneuronal synapses, all the postsynaptic membranes in human beings are chemosensitive.

250 Neuronal transmission at interneuronal synapses occurs in a chemical form.

251 Axon-axonic synapses are the anatomical substrates of presynaptic inhibition.

252 Interneuronal synapses act as two-way valves for propagation of nerve impulses.

253 With reference to interneuronal synapses, the subsynaptic membrane is usually thicker than non-synaptic areas of the postsynaptic membrane.

[Answers on page 127]

Psychopharmacology

254 Droperidol is an example of a thioxanthene.

255 Pimozide is an example of a diphenylbutylpiperidine.

256 Clozapine is an example of a dibenzoxazepine.

257   Prochlorperazine is an example of a phenothiazine.

258   Risperidone is an example of a butyrophenone.

[Answers on page 128]

Pharmacokinetics

259   The placebo effect entails making the patient feel as much at ease as possible.

260   Being married is a predictor of a good response to lithium.

261   An episodic sequence of depression followed by mania is a predictor of a good response to lithium.

262   A response to dexamethasone suppression test is a predictor of a good response to lithium.

263   Lithium concentration in breast milk is approximately 90 per cent of maternal serum concentration.

264   According to current scientific knowledge regarding dopamine receptor subtypes, D_1 receptors are concentrated in the hippocampus.

265   According to current scientific knowledge regarding dopamine receptor subtypes, D_4 receptors are relatively localized to mesolimbic and mesocortical tracts.

266   According to current scientific knowledge regarding dopamine receptor subtypes, D_3 receptors have a distinct regional localization in the limbic system.

267   According to current scientific knowledge regarding dopamine receptor subtypes, clozapine has a tenfold higher affinity for D_4 than D_2 receptors.

268   The dopamine hypothesis of schizophrenia is supported by finding a poor correlation between dopamine blockade and clinical response.

269   The dopamine hypothesis of schizophrenia is not supported by positron emission tomography (PET) studies, which fail to show any difference between untreated patients and normal controls.

270   The dopamine hypothesis of schizophrenia is supported by the fact that negative symptoms markedly improve with dopamine blockade.

271   As regards the pharmacokinetics of antipsychotic drugs, PET studies have shown 40 per cent occupancy of brain D_2 receptors after therapeutic doses.

272   Intramuscular doses of chlorpromazine lead to twofold higher serum levels than corresponding oral doses.

273   About 40 per cent of non-responders are poor absorbers of oral chlorpromazine.

274   Plasma levels of antipsychotic drugs correlate well with plasma prolactin levels.

275   Haloperidol has a high therapeutic index.

276   Concomitant administration of chlorpromazine increases the plasma concentration of lofepramine.

277   Concomitant administration of risperidone increases the plasma concentration of dothiepin.

278   Concomitant administration of carbamazepine reduces the plasma level of amitriptyline.

[Answers on page 128]

Pharmacodynamics

279   Concerning the drug activity and neuroreceptors, drugs that bind to the receptors and initiate a response are called agonists.

280   Drugs that produce a response opposite to the normal response after binding to receptors are called antagonists.

281   Some drugs are known to have both agonistic and antagonistic activity.

282   Reverse agonists are drugs that produce effects by preventing an agonist from initiating a response.

283   Concerning drug activity and neuroreceptors, an affinity refers to the ease with which a drug attaches to a receptor.

284   Stimulation of dopamine receptors characteristically causes tardive dyskinesia.

285   Stimulation of dopamine receptors characteristically causes acute dystonic reactions.

286   Stimulation of dopamine receptors characteristically causes sedation.

287   Stimulation of dopamine receptors characteristically causes nausea and vomiting.

288   Stimulation of dopamine receptors characteristically causes excitement.

289   According to current knowledge about dopamine receptors, D_2 receptors are coupled to adenylate cyclase.

290   According to current knowledge about dopamine receptors, two forms of D_2 receptors have been identified.

291   According to current knowledge about dopamine receptors, D_3 and D_4 receptors have also been identified.

292   According to current knowledge about dopamine receptors, D_2 receptors are coupled with G-proteins.

293   According to current knowledge about dopamine receptors, D_1 receptors are found in abundance in the pituitary gland.

294   Opioids cause constipation by inducing spasm of the stomach and intestines.

295   Tolerance to lysergic acid diethylamide (LSD) usually occurs after three or four daily doses.

296   Anxiety is the commonest feature of an abrupt withdrawal of LSD.

297   Phencyclidine (PCP) exhibits a neuroprotective effect against nerve cell damage arising from cerebral hypoxia.

298   Cross-tolerance occurs between cannabinoids and psychomimetic drugs.

299   Benzodiazepines interact with alpha-adrenergic blockers leading to an enhanced hypotensive effect.

300   Plasma concentration of cimetidine increases when combined with tricyclic antidepressant drugs.

301   The antidepressant action of a psychotropic drug is due to blockade of postsynaptic reuptake of 5-hydroxytryptamine.

302   The antidepressant action of a psychotropic drug is due to downregulation of beta-adrenergic receptors.

303   The antidepressant action of a psychotropic drug is due to blockade of presynaptic reuptake of noradrenaline.

304   The antidepressant action of a psychotropic drug is due to blockade of postsynaptic reuptake of dopamine.

305   The antidepressant action of a psychotropic drug is due to inhibition of synaptic monoamine oxidases.

306   High molecular weight of a psychotropic drug enhances its passage through the blood–brain barrier.

307   Active metabolites of a psychotropic drug enhance its passage through the blood–brain barrier.

308   Low protein binding of a psychotropic drug enhances its passage through the blood–brain barrier.

309   High lipid solubility of a psychotropic drug enhances its passage through the blood–brain barrier.

310   A psychotropic drug enhances its passage through the blood–brain barrier by avoiding first bypass in the liver.

[Answers on page 128]

Adverse drug reactions

311 Lithium-induced neurotoxicity can occur during maintenance therapy.

312 Lithium-induced neurotoxicity can occur despite the serum lithium level being within the therapeutic range.

313 Lithium-induced neurotoxicity is usually precipitated by restricted fluid intake.

314 Lithium-induced neurotoxicity results in persisting neurological sequelae in some patients.

315 Lithium-induced neurotoxicity leads to unique electroencephalographic changes.

316 Anterograde amnesia is a recognized side effect of benzodiazepines in therapeutic doses.

317 Ataxia is a recognized side effect of benzodiazepines in therapeutic doses.

318 Blurred vision is a recognized side effect of benzodiazepines in therapeutic doses.

319 Maculopapular rashes are a recognized side effect of benzodiazepines in therapeutic doses.

320 Nausea is a recognized side effect of benzodiazepines in therapeutic doses.

321 Anorgasmia as a side effect of selective serotonin reuptake inhibitors may be treated with a 5-hydroxytryptamine blocker.

322 Excessive sweating associated with tricyclic antidepressant drugs may be treated with an alpha-1 blocker.

323 Polyuria associated with lithium may be treated with carbamazepine.

324 Leucopenia associated with carbamazepine may be treated with lithium.

325 Impaired ejaculation associated with tricyclic antidepressant drugs may be treated with neostigmine.

326 Hyponatraemia is associated with all types of antidepressant drugs.

327 Neuroleptic malignant syndrome may arise in the course of antidepressant drug treatment.

328 History of epilepsy is an absolute contraindication for the use of clozapine.

[Answers on page 129]

Drug dependence

329   Increased sensory perception is a characteristic feature of benzodiazepine withdrawal syndrome.

330   Anxiety is a characteristic feature of benzodiazepine withdrawal syndrome.

331   Headache is a characteristic feature of benzodiazepine withdrawal syndrome.

332   Depersonalization is a characteristic feature of benzodiazepine withdrawal syndrome.

333   Anorexia is a characteristic feature of benzodiazepine withdrawal syndrome.

[Answers on page 130]

Genetics

334   According to current scientific knowledge, cerebellar ataxia occurs only in males.

335   According to current scientific knowledge, phenylketonuria occurs only in males.

336   According to current scientific knowledge, Gaucher's disease occurs only in males.

337   According to current scientific knowledge, X-linked hydrocephalus occurs only in males.

338   According to current scientific knowledge, the W syndrome occurs only in males.

339   Laboratory diagnosis of XXY syndrome can be made by examination of a buccal smear for sex chromatin (Barr bodies).

340   Laboratory diagnosis of XYY syndrome can be made by examination of a buccal smear for sex chromatin (Barr bodies).

341   Laboratory diagnosis of Wilson's disease can be made by examination of a buccal smear for sex chromatin (Barr bodies).

342   Laboratory diagnosis of Hartnup's disease can be made by examination of a buccal smear for sex chromatin (Barr bodies).

343   Laboratory diagnosis of Edward's syndrome can be made by examination of buccal smear for sex chromatin (Barr bodies).

344   According to current scientific knowledge, fragile X syndrome is transmitted by a single recessive gene.

345   According to current scientific knowledge, a single recessive gene is responsible for the transmission of the Lesch–Nyhan syndrome.

346   According to current scientific knowledge, the Coffin–Lowry syndrome is transmitted by a single recessive gene.

347   According to current scientific knowledge, a single recessive gene transmits bipolar affective disorder.

348   According to current scientific knowledge, Patau's syndrome is transmitted by a single recessive gene.

349   It is possible to make a prenatal diagnosis of Hunter's syndrome.

350   It is possible to make a prenatal diagnosis of Wilson's hepatolenticular degeneration.

351   It is possible to make a prenatal diagnosis of Tay–Sachs disease.

352   It is possible to make a prenatal diagnosis of Krabbe's disease.

353   It is possible to make a prenatal diagnosis of Niemann–Pick disease.

[Answers on page 130]

Epidemiology

354   As regards matching in epidemiological studies, the comparison group does not usually differ from the study group with regard to the diagnosis.

355   As regards matching in epidemiological studies, the comparison group is matched according to the main features of the study group.

356   As regards matching in epidemiological studies, the matched group eliminates unwanted variables.

357   As regards matching in epidemiological studies, the matched group can eliminate more variables than the investigator intends.

358   As regards matching in epidemiological studies, the matched group is normally a random sample from the population from which it is drawn.

[Answers on page 130]

Statistics and research methodology

359   A statistically significant association at $P=0.05$ between two variables implies that a cause and effect relation is established.

360   A statistically significant association at $P=0.05$ between two variables implies that approximately 95 per cent of the variance has been accounted for in the particular experiment.

361 A statistically significant association at $P=0.05$ between two variables implies that an association is likely to occur by chance only in 5/100 cases.

362 A statistically significant association at $P=0.05$ between two variables implies that measurements are of proved validity and reliability.

363 A statistically significant association at $P=0.05$ between two variables implies that the data are trustworthy and useful.

364 The standard error is a measure of central tendency.

365 The standard error is a measure of the most frequent observation.

366 The standard error is a measure of range of observations.

367 The standard error is a measure of the mean of the population.

368 The standard error is a measure of robustness of the experiment.

369 Median is a measure of central tendency of distribution.

370 Mode is a measure of central tendency of distribution.

371 Average is a measure of central tendency of distribution.

372 Quartiles are measures of central tendency of distribution.

373 Range is a measure of central tendency of distribution.

374 Statistically significant association between two variables implies that the association is likely to occur by chance only at a stated low level of probability.

375 Statistically significant association between two variables implies that the P value is >0.001.

376 The characteristic features of Poisson's distribution include a unimodal type of distribution.

377 Poisson's distribution requires events to occur randomly in space or time.

378 In Poisson's distribution, the mean number of events per given unit of time or space is constant.

379 Poisson's distribution requires the events to occur simultaneously.

380 In Poisson's distribution, the sum of corresponding probabilities is one.

381 Cohort studies include defined groups of individuals studied over a period of time.

382 Cohort studies can only be conducted as prospective studies.

383 Cohort studies include changes in the population due to age, which must be distinguished from the disease process.

384   Period effects affect the cohort studies.

385   Cohort studies provide valuable information on the nature of a relationship between two groups.

386   The geometric mean is the reciprocal of the harmonic mean.

387   The geometric mean is the square root of the products of more than two observations.

388   The geometric mean should be used in preference to the arithmetic mean in dealing with sensitive data.

389   The geometric mean is computed by dividing the coefficient of variance by the standard deviation.

390   The geometric mean is a better representative than the arithmetic mean in skewed observations.

391   Quality of life year (QALY) is a useful and acceptable outcome measurement for use in elderly patients.

392   Clifton Assessment Procedures for the Elderly (CAPE-BRS) is a useful and acceptable outcome measurement instrument for use in elderly patients.

393   Health of the Nation Outcome Scales is a useful and acceptable measurement tool for use in elderly patients.

394   Camberwell Assessment of Need for the Elderly is a useful and acceptable measurement tool for use in elderly patients.

[Answers on page 131]

Medical ethics and principles of law

395   The Declaration of Geneva (World Medical Association) has adopted a replacement of the Hippocratic Oath in the UK.

396   The Declaration of Hawaii (World Psychiatric Association, 1977) is one of the best known psychiatric codes available.

397   With reference to deontology (absolutism), rights and duties determine action.

398   With reference to deontology (absolutism), there are procedures to resolve conflicts of rights.

399   With reference to teleology (utilitarianism/consequentialism), the greatest good of the greatest number determines action.

400   Teleology (utilitarianism/consequentialism) relies heavily on rule based assumptions.

[Answers on page 131]

Answers

Psychology

Basic, behavioural and social psychology

1   True
2   True
3   False
4   False
5   True   Drive reduction theory suggests that most people avoid extreme tension-producing situations, but that some seek out such situations. Biological homoeostasis and physiological homoeostasis are associated with the intrinsic theory of motivation.
6   False
7   True
8   False
9   True
10   False

Neuropsychology

11   True
12   True
13   False
14   True
15   True

Human development

16   True
17   False   It is related to fixation in the anal phase.
18   True
19   True
20   False   Eric Erikson described this as a defect due to failure to resolve adolescent issues.
21   False   It is a manifestation of attachment between infant and mother.
22   True   It usually occurs between 3 and 6 years of age.
23   True   It usually occurs between 6 and 12 years of age.
24   False   It is the second stage of cognitive development of the child, as proposed by Piaget.
25   True   It occurs between 12 and 18 years of age.
26   True
27   False   The concrete operational stage is associated with mastery of conservation.
28   True

29   **False**   The formal operational stage is associated with the ability to detach logic from immediate experience.

30   **True**

31   **True**

32   **False**

33   **True**

34   **False**

35   **True**   Maslow's unified theory describes a hierarchy of needs, ranked according to survival importance. It includes physical safety and self-actualization.

36   **False**

37   **False**   Adolescent turmoil is considered inevitable and beneficial. It probably arises due to stress in dealing with various developmental tasks of adolescence.

38   **False**

39   **True**

40   **True**

Assessment, description and measurement of behaviour

41   **False**

42   **False**

43   **True**

44   **True**

45   **False**   Maguire and Rutter (1976)* found that final year medical students were deficient in psychiatric interviewing techniques. Personal areas of the history were avoided, and if the patient volunteered these topics, the student would shift the interview to more neutral topics. *Maguire GP, Rutter DR (1976) History taking for medical students. I Deficiencies in performance. *Lancet* ii: 556–8.

46   **True**

47   **False**

48   **False**

49   **False**

50   **True**   The Present State Examination provides criteria for severity as well, since it assesses the patient's mental state at the time of interview and in the previous month. Information about past illness is not obtained. The Schedule for Affective Disorders and Schizophrenia is a widely used interview schedule in the USA. It covers a wide range of conditions including personality disorders and alcohol-related syndromes, unlike the Present State Examination.

51   **False**

52   **False**

53   **True**   In the Thurstone scale, the subject is presented with a range of statements, in which the subject ticks those with which he or she agrees. The Likert scale is a 5-point scale.

54   **True**
55   **True**

Basis of psychological treatments

56   **True**
57   **False**
58   **False**
59   **False**
60   **False**

Social sciences and ethology

61   **True**
62   **True**
63   **True**
64   **False**   More often found in neurotic patients.
65   **True**
66   **False**
67   **False**
68   **False**
69   **True**
70   **True**
71   **True**
72   **True**
73   **True**
74   **False**
75   **True**   According to Festinger's theory of cognitive dissonance, the more important the cognitions, the more powerful the dissonance.
76   **True**
77   **True**
78   **True**
79   **False**   Type A personality tends to be associated with an increased rate of myocardial infarction and angina pectoris.
80   **True**
81   **True**
82   **True**
83   **True**   Fixed action pattern is a genetically established sequence of motor activity that is triggered by a sign stimulus to release the particular pattern of behaviour.
84   **False**   Ethnic bonds appear to be learned rather than biologically determined.
85   **True**

Neurosciences

Neuroanatomy

86 True

87 True

88 True

89 False   Oligodendrocytes form the myelin sheaths of central neurones. Schwann cells form the myelin sheaths of peripheral neurones.

90 True

91 True

92 False

93 False

94 False

95 True

96 True   The optic nerve is the sensory nerve of the retina. The optic chiasma is situated medial to the internal carotid arteries.

97 False

98 False

99 True

100 True

101 True

102 False   Occlusion of the anterior cerebral artery results in contralateral hemiparesis, affecting the lower limbs more than the upper limbs.

103 True

104 True

105 True

106 False   It consists of three layers.

107 True

108 True   Pyramidal cells, stellate cells, multiform cells, cells of Martinotti and the horizontal cells of Cajal.

109 False   It is a part of the archicortex.

110 False   They form the most superficial layer.

111 False

112 True

113 False

114 False   The auditory cortex receives information from both ears because the auditory pathway is not entirely crossed.

115 True

116 True   Primary association areas are adjacent to the sensory area and give rise to projections, which are more widespread, called secondary association areas.

117 True

118 False   The primary sensory cortex receives input from the relay nuclei of the thalamus.

119 True

120 **True**

121 **True**

122 **False** The afferent fibres bypass the lateral geniculate bodies and pass medially to the superior colliculi.

123 **True**

124 **False** The afferent fibres never reach the occipital cortex but end in the occulomotor nuclei, from where the efferent path originates.

125 **True**

126 **False** Mitochondria are present throughout the neurone and are involved in energy production. Dendrites also contain Nissl substance, which synthesizes proteins.

127 **False** Dendrites, like the cell body and axon hillock of the neurone, are unmyelinated.

128 **False** They are found in both the central nervous system (brain and spinal cord) and the peripheral nervous system (cranial and spinal nerves and other neuronal processes).

129 **True** The dendritic spines form the subsynaptic membrane (synaptic plates) of the axodendritic synapses.

130 **True**

131 **False**

132 **False**

133 **False**

134 **False**

135 **False** The dopamine containing fibres originate in nucleus A10 and innervate the olfactory tubercle, septal nuclei (lateral septal nucleus and nucleus accumbens), interstitial cells of the stria terminalis, cingulate cortex and the oval part of the parahippocampal cortex.

Neuropathology

136 **False** The plaques consist of amyloid precursor protein deposits surrounded by astrocytic and microglial cells.

137 **False** The neurofibrillary tangles are paired helical filaments.

138 **True**

139 **True**

140 **False** Amyloid deposition occurs in blood vessels.

141 **True**

142 **True**

143 **True**

144 **True**

145 **True**

146 **True**

147 **True**

148 **False** White matter changes, as seen on MRI scan, also occur away from the ventricles and in postmortem studies. These lesions correspond to multiple sclerosis plaques.

149 **True**

150 **True**

151 **True** It consists of numerous microcystic spaces scattered throughout the grey matter, giving the brain a spongy appearance.

152 **True**

153 **False** This pathological feature is found in Wernicke–Korsakoff syndrome.

154 **True**

155 **False** They are present in the basal ganglia and substantia nigra of patients with Parkinson's disease. They have also been found in dementia of Lewy body type.

Neurophysiology

156 **True**

157 **False** Stria terminalis is not considered part of the limbic system.

158 **True**

159 **True**

160 **True**

161 **True**

162 **True**

163 **True**

164 **True**

165 **True**

166 **False**

167 **False**

168 **True** The primary source of energy for the brain is glucose. Unlike other tissues, the brain cannot use lipids and proteins for energy. The brain has little glycogen storage. It can use some ketone bodies when their level is high.

169 **True**

170 **True**

171 **True**

172 **False** 80 per cent of growth hormone is secreted during slow-wave sleep.

173 **True**

174 **True**

175 **True**

176 **False**

177 **False** Lipid-soluble substances pass readily into the brain, as opposed to proteins, which enter more slowly.

178 **True** It regulates the movement of substances into and out of the nervous system.

179 **False**

180 **True** The blood–brain barrier separates the brain and cerebrospinal fluid from the blood. It is represented structurally by the capillary endothelium of the brain, the subarachnoid space and the arachnoid membrane. The cells are tightly bound together.

181 **False**

182 **True**

183 **False**

184 **True**   Lipid-soluble substances pass readily through the blood–brain barrier, whereas non-lipid soluble substances and proteins enter the brain slowly.

185 **True**   This states that the permeability of a cell membrane to a drug is proportional to the drug's partition parameter. The latter is the product of two fractional concentrations, one of the un-ionized drugs in aqueous solution and the other lipid solubility of the un-ionized drug.

186 **False**   It is similar to that of the relaxed wakeful state.

187 **False**   Maturation both in the fetus and throughout life leads to electroencephalogram frequency and wave form changes.

188 **False**   The electroencephalographic changes are similar to those observed with tricyclic antidepressants, such as slowing of the alpha wave and increasing slow wave activity.

189 **True**

190 **True**

191 **True**

192 **False**   Such an activity is a normal feature of sleep.

193 **True**   Alpha rhythm is attenuated by attention and accentuated by eye closure.

194 **True**

195 **False**   In humans, electroencephalographic rhythms vary with age.

196 **True**

197 **False**   Decreased activity is seen but no changes in anatomical size of medial prefrontal cortex.

198 **True**

199 **True**

200 **True**

201 **True**

202 **False**

203 **False**

204 **True**

205 **False**

206 **True**

207 **True**

208 **True**

209 **True**

210 **False**

211 **True**

212 **True**

213 **True**

Neuroendocrinology

214 **False**   Decreased plasma osmolality leads to release of these hormones.

215 **False**   There is a nocturnal surge during slow-wave (stages 3 and 4) sleep.

216 **False**   Usually higher.

217 **True** Noradrenaline and its metabolites (except 3-methoxy-4-hydroxyphenylglycol (MHPG)) do not cross the blood–brain barrier.

218 **True** This may explain the patients' preoccupation with weight loss.

Neurochemistry

219 **True**

220 **True**

221 **True**

222 **True**

223 **True** They cause depolarization of neurones.

224 **False** It is an amino acid.

225 **True** Other monoamines include noradrenaline, adrenaline and serotonin.

226 **False** See answer 224.

227 **True**

228 **False** See answer 224.

229 **True**

230 **False** They are closely associated with K^+ channels and are regulated by gallamine and guanosine triphosphate, and inhibit adenyl cyclase.

231 **True**

232 **False** They are, in fact, nicotine receptor antagonists.

233 **True** They cause confusion, lassitude and drowsiness; and dry mouth, excessive sweating, blurring of vision and urinary retention, respectively.

234 **True**

235 **True**

236 **False** There is no convincing evidence to suggest an increase in dopamine metabolites in the cerebrospinal fluid of patients with schizophrenia.

237 **False** Oral dopamine is absorbed in the gastrointestinal tract.

238 **True**

239 **True**

240 **False** L-Dopa is a dopamine agonist used for the treatment of Parkinson's disease.

241 **True**

242 **True**

243 **True**

244 **True**

245 **True**

246 **True**

247 **True**

248 **False** G-proteins interact with multiple effectors.

249 **True**

250 **False** It involves alternating translations of electrical signals into chemical messages through neurotransmitters and of chemical messages into electrical signals.

251 **True**

252 **False** The synapse acts as a one-way valve, allowing transmission of nerve impulses in one direction only.

253 **True**

Psychopharmacology

254 **False**   Droperidol is a butyrophenone.

255 **True**

256 **False**   Clozapine is a dibenzodiazepine. Loxapine is a dibenzoxazepine.

257 **True**

258 **False**   Risperidone is a benzisoxazole.

Pharmacokinetics

259 **False**

260 **False**

261 **False**   It is the other way round, i.e. mania followed by depression.

262 **False**

263 **False**   About 30 per cent.

264 **False** D_1 receptors are found in caudate nucleus, putamen, nucleus accumbens and olfactory tubercle. D_5 receptors are found in the hippocampus and hypothalamus.

265 **True**   Also in medulla oblongata, midbrain and frontal cortex.

266 **True**

267 **True**

268 **False**

269 **True**

270 **False**   Negative symptoms are minimally improved with dopamine blockade.

271 **False**   65–90 per cent occupancy of D_2 receptors. It appears that receptor occupancy above 70 per cent is necessary for antipsychotic response.

272 **False**   Fourfold or even higher serum levels.

273 **True**   Because of its metabolism to inactive substances in the intestinal wall. Active metabolites are formed in the liver.

274 **True**   Plasma antipsychotic levels correlate with adverse effects and some electroencephalographic changes, such as increases in delta and theta activities. They do not correlate with clinical response.

275 **False**   Haloperidol has a low therapeutic index, i.e. the dose at which the first signs of extrapyramidal side effects (EPS) appear is very close to the required dose for optimum antipsychotic effect in most patients.

276 **True**

277 **True**

278 **True**

Pharmacodynamics

279 **True**   They bind to receptors and initiate a response in neuroeffector tissues.

280 **False**   They prevent an agonist initiating a response.

281 **True**

282 **False**   These are antagonists.
283 **True**
284 **False**
285 **True**   Effect on nigrostriatal pathway
286 **False**   Effect on histamine receptors causes sedation.
287 **False** H_3 antagonism causes nausea and vomiting.
288 **False**
289 **True**
290 **True** D_2 has two isoforms.
291 **True** D_1, D_2, D_3, D_4 and D_5.
292 **True** D_1–D_5 are all G-protein coupled.
293 **False**   Abundant in nucleus accumbens, olfactory tubercles, caudate nucleus and putamen.
294 **True**   Presumably by stimulation of opioid receptors in the myentric plexus.
295 **True**   Due to desensitization of the 5-hydroxytryptamine 2 (5-HT$_2$) receptors.
296 **False**   No noticeable physical or psychological effects on abrupt withdrawal.
297 **True**
298 **False**   Between THC and alcohol.
299 **True**
300 **False**   Increased plasma concentration of tricyclic antidepressant drugs.
301 **False**
302 **False**
303 **True**
304 **False**
305 **True**
306 **False**
307 **False**
308 **False**
309 **True**
310 **False**
311 **True**
312 **True**
313 **False**   Restriction of fluid intake may lead to neurotoxicity.
314 **True**
315 **False**   There are no specific electroencephalographic changes. Increasing episodes of intermittent, high-amplitude diffuse delta waves may be present.
316 **True**   Anterograde amnesia is particularly associated with high potency drugs.
317 **True**
318 **True**
319 **False**   Maculopapular rashes are rare allergic reactions.
320 **True**

321 **True** e.g. cyproheptadine.
322 **True** terazosin.
323 **True** Carbamazepine is an antidiuretic hormone sensitizer.
324 **True**
325 **True**
326 **True**
327 **True**
328 **False**

Drug dependence

329 **True**
330 **True**
331 **True**
332 **True**
333 **True**

Genetics

334 **True**
335 **False** Autosomal recessive disorder of protein metabolism.
336 **False** Autosomal recessive disorder of lipid metabolism.
337 **True**
338 **True**
339 **True** One extra X chromosome and one Barr body.
340 **False** One extra Y chromosome and no Barr body.
341 **False** It is an autosomal recessive disorder of copper metabolism.
342 **False** Autosomal recessive disorder of protein metabolism.
343 **False** Trisomy 18.
344 **False**
345 **False** Fragile X syndrome and Lesch–Nyhan syndrome are X-linked recessive disorders.
346 **False** X-linked dominant disorder.
347 **False** Does not follow Mendelian inheritance.
348 **False** Trisomy 13.
349 **False** A defect of iduronate sulphatase.
350 **False** Defect of copper metabolism.
351 **True** A defect of hexosaminidase A (fat metabolism).
352 **True** A defect of galactocerebroside.
353 **False** A defect of sphingomyelinase (fat metabolism).

Epidemiology

354 **False**
355 **True**
356 **True**
357 **True**
358 **False**

Statistics and research methodology

359 **True**   The establishment of a cause and effect relation requires a different procedure.
360 **True**
361 **True**
362 **False**   Different procedures are required to establish validity and reliability.
363 **True**
364 **False**
365 **False**
366 **False**
367 **True**
368 **True**   The standard error is a measure of how much variation in test results is due to chance and error and how much is due to experimental influences.
369 **True**
370 **True**
371 **True**
372 **False**   They measure values other than central tendency.
373 **False**
374 **True**
375 **False** $P<0.001$ indicates a statistically highly significant association.
376 **False**   It is a bimodal type of distribution.
377 **True**
378 **True**
379 **False**   In fact, it requires events to be independent.
380 **True**
381 **True**
382 **False**   They can be retrospective as well.
383 **True**
384 **True**
385 **True**
386 **False**
387 **True**
388 **False**
389 **False**
390 **True**
391 **False**
392 **True**
393 **True**
394 **True**

Medical ethics and principles of law

395 **False**   The Declaration of Geneva is of little value in guiding particular clinical decisions.

396 **True** The other one is Principles of Medical Ethics with annotations especially applicable to psychiatry (American Psychiatric Association, 1973)†. However, its principles are set forth as an unargued list. †American Psychiatric Association (1973) (revised 1988) *Principles of Medical Ethics with Annotations Especially Applicable to Psychiatry.* APA, Washington DC.

397 **True**

398 **False** No procedures are available.

399 **True**

400 **False** Teleology relies heavily on the assumption that it is possible to measure various possible outcomes of moral choices in terms of pleasure or pain, happiness lost or gained for all those affected.

11 BASIC SCIENCES: PAPER 4 (EMIs)

Note: In EMIs each option may be used once, more than once or not at all.

Sample questions

1 Differential diagnosis of genetic disorders

A Angelman's syndrome
B Asperger's syndrome
C Fragile X syndrome
D Joubert's syndrome
E Lesch–Nyhan syndrome
F Prader–Willi syndrome
G Rett's syndrome
H Turner's syndrome

Select one option from the list above for the following clinical scenarios.

1 A 12-year-old boy is brought to the outpatient clinic by his parents as they are very concerned about him. He has always been a loner. He has been having problems at school recently. He is being bullied very often as he tends to do solitary activities at school. On examination, there is no evidence of learning disability or speech delay. He has a special interest in maps and has a number of books on them.

2 A 15-year-old male boy with learning disability is brought to the accident and emergency department by his parents following a seizure. On examination he appears to be very shy and avoids eye contact. He also has microcephaly and macro-orchidism.

3 The parents of a 5-year-old boy bring him to the outpatient clinic as they are worried about his health. He had been eating a lot resulting in excessive weight gain. He has mild learning disability. It was noted that he tended to pick his skin repeatedly and this often causes bleeding.

[Answers on page 166]

2 Genetics of organic brain disorders

A 25 per cent of the children affected
B Autosomal dominant transmission
C Autosomal recessive transmission
D Chromosome 5
E Chromosome 11
F Chromosome 20
G Mutations in the *tau* gene
H Sex-linked dominant transmission
I Sex-linked recessive transmission

For each of the following vignettes choose one option from the list above which best describes the vignette.

1   A 2-year-old girl was brought to the outpatient clinic by her parents. She used to be a happy and cheerful child until she had a seizure a month ago. Since then she has not been able to walk properly and has also stopped talking. They have noticed repeated hand-wringing movements.

2   A 5-year-old boy was brought to the outpatient clinic by his parents who are very worried about him. He has a diagnosis of learning disability. He has recently started showing self-injurious behaviour in the form of biting himself and banging his head. On examination he has spasticity, ataxia and choreoathetoid movements.

3   The parents of a 3-year-old girl bring her to the accident and emergency department following a seizure. She has facial angiofibroma and hypopigmented irises. She was fine until recently.

[Answers on page 166]

3 Differential diagnosis of patients with learning disability

A Asperger's syndrome
B Down's syndrome
C Fragile X syndrome
D Infantile autism
E Lawrence–Moon–Biedl syndrome
F Marfan's syndrome
G Smith–Magenis syndrome
H Williams' syndrome

For each of the following vignettes choose one option from the list above which best describes the vignette.

1   A 19-year-old man presents with dysmorphic features and borderline intellectual functioning. On examination, he displays good language abilities but prominent deficits in visuomotor integration.

2   The parents of a 4-year-old boy are concerned that their son has delayed acquisition of speech, reduced or no eye contact and displays repetitive stereotyped behaviour. He does not mix with other children and looks happy on his own.

3   An 8-year-old boy is referred to the outpatient clinic with history of moderate learning disability, poor attention, overeating, bruxism and self-injurious behaviour. On examination, he has both conductive and sensorimotor deafness and stereotyped hand movements.

[Answers on page 166]

4 Clinicopathological correlations of dementia

A Atrophy of the frontal poles
B Degeneration of the mediodorsal thalamic nucleus
C Intraneuronal deposits of ubiquitinated neurofilaments in the cortex and substantia nigra
D Mutation in presenilin-1 (*PS1*) gene
E Mutation in the *tau* gene
F Neurofibrillary tangles and amyloid plaques in the neocortex
G Presence of epsilon 4 (*E4*) allele of the apolipoprotein E (*apoE*) gene
H Sensitivity to antipsychotic drugs
I Thiamine deficiency

For each of the following choose the most appropriate options from the list above. Follow the instruction given after each question.

1 A 62-year-old married woman presents with a history of altered behaviour, disinhibition and apathy of several months' duration. On examination, she is mildly disorientated in time, place and person. Her mother and a maternal aunt had a similar condition. (Choose the two best options.)

2 A 75-year-old man presents with a history of progressive dementia and dysphasia. His dementia began with memory loss for recent events but has now become more generalized. He had a head injury with loss of consciousness 20 years ago, and has history of alcohol misuse. (Choose the two best options.)

3 A 73-year-old woman presents with a history of visual hallucinations, parkinsonism and fluctuating confusion. (Choose the two best options.)

[Answers on page 166]

5 Behavioural genetics and phenotypes of mental disorders

A Autism
B Ataxia
C Cerebral gigantism
D Hair pulling
E Hand-wringing movements
F Impulsive eating
G Learning disability
H Psychopathy
I Repeated self-injuries
J Social anxiety
K Under-developed genitalia

For each of the following vignettes choose options from the list above. Follow the instruction given after each question.

1   A 2-year-old girl previously healthy is brought to the outpatient clinic by her mother who is worried about her. She is no longer able to say the words she learnt previously and has had seizures. (Choose the two best options.)

2   A 12-year-old boy repeatedly picks at his skin. He is obese and tends to overeat and has been diagnosed with cardiac problems. (Choose the three best options.)

3   A 20-year-old man is brought by police as he assaulted someone in a pub following an argument. He has mild learning disability and the secondary sexual characters are not well developed. He has gynaecomastia. He went to a state school and left at 16 without any qualification. (Choose the two best options.)

[Answers on page 137]

6 Mechanism of action of psychoactive chemical substances

A Caffeine
B Cholecystokinin
C Clonidine
D Fenfluramine
E Flumazenil
F Gamma-aminobutyric acid (GABA)
G Nortriptyline
H Reboxetine
I Selegiline
J Sertraline

For each of the following choose the most appropriate option from the list above.

1   This drug has been used to treat multidrug-resistant depression in Parkinson's disease. It has no dopaminergic, histamine, adrenergic or serotonergic effects, and acts mainly on the noradrenergic system.

2   Sudden withdrawal of this drug can cause headaches, rebound drowsiness, fatigue, lethargy and depression. This drug has been used intravenously to augment seizure duration during electroconvulsive therapy.

3   This drug is useful in blocking the noradrenergic aspects of anxiety but is less powerful in blocking the subjective/emotional aspects of anxiety. The same properties of the drug make it quite useful in detoxification from alcohol and sedatives.

[Answers on page 166]

7 Mechanism of action of adverse effects of psychotropic drugs

A Alpha-1 adrenergic receptor
B Alpha-2 adrenergic receptor
C Dopamine D_2 receptor
D Gamma-aminobutyric acid (GABA) receptor
E Histamine H_1 receptor
F 5-Hydroxytryptamine 2C (5-HT_{2C}) receptor
G Mu receptor
H Sigma receptor

For each of the following vignettes choose one option from the list above that explains the underlying mechanism of action in each vignette.

1   A 30-year-old single, unemployed man develops opiate dependence.

2   A 29-year-old married woman suffers from treatment-resistant schizophrenia. Her weight increases significantly after 6 months of treatment with clozapine.

3   A 19-year-old single man was admitted to a psychiatric ward following an acute psychotic breakdown. He was treated with chlorpromazine for 2 days. He complains of daytime drowsiness.

[Answers on page 167]

8 Mechanism of action of psychotropic drugs

A Amitriptyline
B Cocaine
C Desipramine
D Glycine
E Ketamine
F Mirtazapine
G Ondansetron
H PCP (phencyclidine)
I Ritanserin
J Tetrabenazine

For each of the following types of action, select the most appropriate options from the list above. Follow the instruction given after each action.

1   N-methyl-D-aspartate (NMDA) antagonism. (Choose the two best options.)

2   Reuptake inhibitions of neurotransmitters. (Choose the three best options.)

3   5-Hydroxytryptamine 3 (5-HT$_3$) antagonism. (Choose the two best options.)

[Answers on page 167]

9 Electroencephalographic changes in mental disorders

A Alpha rhythm
B Beta rhythm
C Reduced sleep latency
D Saw-tooth waves
E Spike and slow wave complexes
F 3 H Spike and wave
G 'Spindles'
H Theta rhythms

For each of the following vignettes choose one option from the list above that would occur in the vignette.

1   A 49-year-old married company executive is admitted for assessment of his mental state. He is thought to have a rapid-onset dementia characterized by ataxia and myoclonic jerks.

2   A 37-year-old single male factory worker is admitted to a neurological unit for investigation of 5-year history of undue sleepiness and episodic leg weakness. A diagnosis of narcolepsy is considered.

3   A 62-year-old married man was admitted to a surgical ward following an acute abdomen. Three days after an exploratory surgery, he complained of feeling anxious, shaky and mildly confused. He is experiencing vivid visual hallucinations.

[Answers on page 167]

10 Identification of metabolic/biochemical abnormalities

A Hypercalcaemia
B Hyperglycaemia
C Hypoglycaemia
D Hyperkalaemia
E Hypokalaemia
F Hypernatraemia
G Hyponatraemia
H Hyperthyroidism
I Hypothyroidism

For each of the following case histories choose one option which describes the most likely abnormality that may occur in each patient.

1   A 40-year-old man with a history of alcohol dependence syndrome presents with marked symptoms of anxiety. He had indulged himself in a binge approximately 12 hours ago.

2   A 38-year-old single man with treatment-resistant paranoid schizophrenia presents with increasing behavioural disturbances and mental confusion. He started taking clozapine about 8 weeks ago with beneficial effect.

3   A 60-year-old man suffering from diabetes mellitus presents with lethargy, nausea and muscle cramps for few days. He has a history of depression currently treated with paroxetine and amitriptyline.

[Answers on page 167]

11 Applications of study designs in clinical research

A Case–control study
B Cross-sectional survey
C Economic analysis
D Observational cohort
E Pragmatic trial
F Prospective single case study
G Randomized controlled clinical trial
H Retrospective case–control study

For each of the following studies, select the most appropriate option from the list above.

1   A study is planned to determine the causes of a rare disease in a local population.

2   A study is planned to determine an association between two common diseases.

3   A study is planned to evaluate the efficacy of a new intervention in patients with schizophrenia.

[Answers on page 167]

12 Applications of study designs in clinical research

A Case-control study

B Case series

C Cross-sectional study

D Ecological study

E Observational cohort

F Randomized controlled trial

G Systematic review

H Uncontrolled clinical trial

For each of the following studies, select the most appropriate option from the list above.

1   A study to assess the benefit of a new expensive investigation in the general population.

2   A study is planned to evaluate the occupational hazards of the nuclear industry, and any association between exposure and possible outcomes.

3   A study to assess the efficacy of an experimental, new diagnostic procedure in a given sample.

[Answers on page 167]

13 Applications of multivariate analysis in clinical research

A Analysis of covariance
B Analysis of variance
C Discriminant functional analysis
D Factor analysis
E Kruskal–Wallis analysis of variance
F Log linear modelling
G Mann–Whitney U test
H One-way analysis of variance

For each of the following studies, select the most appropriate option from the list above.

1   A study designed to evaluate the effects of gender, socioeconomic condition and marital status of both men and women.

2   One hundred and fifty patients with mild to moderate diabetes are randomly assigned to one of two treatment options. Blood sugar levels are determined before and after treatment with an interval of 1 month. Effects of both treatments are compared in this study.

3   A study is designed to examine the effects of 21 items of life stressors at 6 months to predict the onset of illness following the health screening.

[Answers on page 167]

14 Applications of multivariate analysis in clinical research

A Analysis of covariance
B Analysis of variance
C Cluster analysis
D Discriminant functional analysis
E Latent trait analysis
F One-way analysis of variance
G Path analysis
H Principal component analysis

For each of the following studies, select the most appropriate options from the list above. Follow the instruction given after each question.

1   It is necessary to determine two indices one measuring demoralization and the other measuring summarization, based on the information obtained from four separate questionnaires administered to 200 people. Those questions were initially devised to assess anxiety, depression, anger and psychopathology. (Choose one best option.)

2   It is suitable for independent measures and repeated measures taken in two or more occasions in the same individuals. (Choose one best option.)

3   It is suitable for identification of groups of variables and their interactions that determine the group status of the subjects. (Choose the two best options.)

[Answers on page 168]

15 Identification of bias in research studies

A Berkson's bias
B Interviewer bias
C No bias
D Overmatching
E Publication bias
F Recall bias
G Selection bias
H Social desirability bias

For each of the following studies, select the most appropriate option from the list above.

1   In a case–control study of toxic shock syndrome, demonstrating that brand A tampons were a cause of the syndrome, the controls were age and race matched. The study used a postal questionnaire.

2   For a study of efficacy of antidepressants, patients were taken from outpatient clinics and were matched according to their age, sex and occupation.

3   In case–control study of the relation between diethylstilbestrol (DES) use during pregnancy and subsequent development of vaginal cancer in the offspring, the controls were chosen from birth records. The controls were the next recorded female birth from the same hospital where the patient was born. The use of DES was ascertained by inspection of medical and obstetric records.

[Answers on page 168]

16 Identification of bias in research studies

A Berkson's bias
B No flaws
C Overmatching
D Publication bias
E Recall bias
F Response bias
G Sampling bias
H Selection bias

For each of the following studies, select the most appropriate option from the list above.

1   In a case–control study of importance of exposure to benzene as a cause of leukaemia, the controls were chosen from among workmates of the cases.

2   To ascertain the efficacy of selective serotonin reuptake inhibitors (SSRIs), all randomized controlled trials were selected from *British Journal of Psychiatry*, *American Journal of Psychiatry*, and publications available in the library of the Royal College of Psychiatrists.

3   An observation that hospitalized schizophrenic patients rarely had epilepsy led to the introduction of electroconvulsive therapy.

[Answers on page 168]

17 Methods of statistical analysis of research data

A Bonferroni's correction
B Chi-squared test
C Correlation coefficient
D Mann–Whitney U test
E Scheffe's test
F Student's paired *t* test
G Student's *t* test
H Wilcoxon's matched-pairs signed rank test

For each of the following studies, select the most appropriate option from the list above.

1   Seventy patients with schizophrenia were randomly assigned to receive treatment A or placebo. They were reassessed after 3 months of treatment and rated as improved, no change or deteriorated.

2   Two surgically similar wounds were inflicted on each rabbit. One wound was sutured while the other was taped. At the end of 10 days tensile strength was measured using a spring scale that was judged to be accurate to about 69 kPa (10 psi).

3   A study is designed to determine whether there is any relation between blood pressure and blood sugar level. Both were measured in a cross-sectional group of hypertensive patients.

[Answers on page 168]

18 Methods of statistical analysis of research data

A Chi-squared test
B Logistic regression
C Multiple regression
D Pearson's correlation coefficient
E Spearman's rank correlation coefficient
F Student's paired t test
G Student's t test
H Wilcoxon's rank sum test

For each of the following studies, select the most appropriate option from the list above.

1   Fifty patients with diabetes mellitus were treated with active drug and placebo for 1 month using a sophisticated crossover design and a washout period. Blood sugar levels were measured during treatment with active drug and placebo according to the protocol.

2   It is useful when the dependent variable is continuous and the interrelationships between variables are linear.

3   It is useful when the dependent variable is binary (dichotomous) and the risk of developing an outcome (or not) is expressed as a function of independent predictor variables.

[Answers on page 168]

19 Determining appropriate controls in research studies

A A gold standard drug
B Community controls
C Healthy controls
D Historical controls
E Hospital controls
F Matched controls
G No control group
H Placebo

For each of the following studies, select the most appropriate options from the list above that fulfil the objectives. Follow the instruction given after each question.

1 A new case–control study of depression is designed to overcome the criticism that previous studies were affected by Berkson's bias. (Choose one best option.)

2 A study is designed to investigate a new treatment for an invariably fatal disease. (Choose the two best options.)

3 A cross-sectional study of incidence and prevalence of bipolar disorder in the general population. (Choose one best option.)

[Answers on page 168]

20 Identification of bias in clinical research studies

A Attrition bias
B Berkson's bias
C Confounding bias
D Membership bias
E Neyman's bias
F Publication bias
G Recall bias
H Selection bias

For each of the following vignettes choose one option from the list above which best describes the vignette.

1   A case–control study is designed to look at the association between the use of illicit drugs and the first episode of psychosis. The subjects with psychosis may be more likely to remember which illicit drugs they have used.

2   A cohort study is looking at the long-term association between regular cannabis use and subsequent occurrence of schizophrenia. It is believed that the subjects in the cannabis group are more likely to drop out on follow-up.

3   In a placebo-controlled trial of a new antipsychotic drug, the group allocation is based on the hospital registration numbers. The investigator who recruits the subjects for the study will know to which treatment group they will be allocated.

[Answers on page 168]

21 Application of tests of statistical analysis

A Analysis of covariance (ANCOVA)
B Analysis of variance (ANOVA)
C Chi-squared test
D Cluster analysis
E Fisher's exact probability test
F Mann–Whitney U test
G Multivariate analysis
H Regression analysis
I Student's paired *t* test
J Student's unpaired *t* test

For each of the following choose options from the list above. Follow the instruction given after each question

1   A study is conducted in a group of individuals who had received a diagnosis of conduct disorder 10 years ago. At the time, their IQ and height were measured which were found to be normally distributed and significantly correlated. Now the sample is assessed for the presence or absence of personality disorder. Which test will be useful to test the hypothesis of relation between IQ and the presence or absence of personality disorder? (Choose the two best options.)

2   In the above sample, it is decided to examine the influence of gender on the likelihood of developing personality disorder. Now which tests would be more suitable? (Choose the two best options.)

3   In the same sample in question, it is decided to examine the influence of height and IQ on the likelihood of developing personality disorder. Which tests should be used now? (Choose the two best options.)

[Answers on page 168]

22 Application of tests of statistical analysis in clinical research

A Canonical correlation
B Chi-squared test
C Cluster analysis
D Factor analysis
E Mann–Whitney U test
F Multivariate analysis of variance (MANOVA)
G One-tailed Student's *t* test
H One-way analysis of variance (ANOVA)
I Regression analysis
J Two-way analysis of variance (ANOVA)

For each of the following, select the most appropriate statistical test from the list above.

1   A study is designed to test the hypothesis that sex and social status of patients, the level of expressed emotion in their family and the type of antipsychotic drug determine relapse rates in schizophrenia. A number of variables are measured in a large group of patients.

2   A study is designed to test the hypothesis that the cortisol response to adrenocorticotropic hormone (ACTH) is increased in depressed patients compared with controls. Plasma cortisol concentrations are measured every 30 minutes, over a 2-hour period following the administration of an intravenous bolus of ACTH.

3   A study is designed to test the hypothesis that atypical antipsychotics lead to a better quality of life compared with typical antipsychotics. A composite score of health status and functional ability assessed independently by both patients and their doctors are to be used to compare the two groups of patients on different treatments.

[Answers on page 169]

23 Clinical application of learning theories

A Cognitive map
B Classical conditioning
C Extinction
D Premack's principle
E Operant conditioning
F Shaping
G Stimulus generalization
H Reciprocal inhibition

For each of the following scenarios, choose one option from the list above that best describes the situation.

1   A 10-year-old boy likes to play football and neglects eating. His parents are advised to allow him to play football only after eating.

2   A 12-year-old girl is bitten by a non-poisonous snake while playing in the garden. Now she is afraid of ropes and refuses to play in the garden.

3   A 12-year-old girl who developed a phobia after being bitten by a non-poisonous snake is exposed to rope repeatedly. Phobic symptoms gradually disappear.

[Answers on page 169]

24 Clinical applications of learning theories

A Cognitive map
B Classical conditioning
C Extinction
D Premack's principle
E Operant conditioning
F Shaping
G Stimulus generalization
H Reciprocal inhibition

For each of the following scenarios choose the most appropriate option from the list above.

1 A bell is rung first before presenting food to a dog for several days. The dog salivates every time the bell rings alone.

2 A 35-year-old man who has developed spider phobia is put into a relaxed state by suggestion and soothing music. He is shown a photograph of a black spider.

3 In order to induce a rat to press a bar, food is given when it approaches the lever. Then food is given when it touches the lever and then when it actually presses the lever.

[Answers on page 169]

25 Identification of the components of cognitive functions

A Dichotic listening
B Divided attention
C Focused attention
D Impaired attention
E Motion parallel
F Perspective cue
G Retinal disparity
H Shadowing
I Split-span experiment
J Sustained attention

For each of the following vignettes choose one option from the list above which best describes the vignette.

1   A 5-year-old boy is looking out of the train window. He appears perplexed and asks his mother why the trees near to him tend to move away fast whereas the trees far away tend to move slowly.

2   A 40-year-old man eats his meal enthusiastically. At the same time he has turned the radio on and is listening to music.

3   A 9-year-old boy has his headphones on. A random number of digits are being spoken in his right ear and a random number of words are spoken in his left ear at the same time. The task for him is to repeat what he hears in his left ear.

[Answers on page 169]

26 Identification of learning theory underlying human behaviour

A Classical conditioning
B Chaining
C Covert sensitization
D Higher-order conditioning
E Punishment
F Shaping
G Stimulus discrimination
H Stimulus generalization

For each of the following choose the most appropriate options from the list above. Follow the instruction given after each question.

1   A family bought a young cat recently. It initially responded to all members of the family and to visitors. However, over time, the cat learnt to respond only to commands of two family members.

2   A 10-year-old boy talks about several topics in presence of his parents. His parents reinforce his behaviour by praising and encouraging him every time he engages in an interesting discussion. The boy is now keen to talk to visitors and teachers.

3   A 4-year-old girl is learning to write. Her parents praise her for holding the pencil correctly and then scribbling something. She keeps trying to write words.

—[Answers on page 169]

27 Understanding human behaviour on the basis of learning theories

A Avoidance learning
B Classical conditioning
C Discriminative learning
D Extinction
E Modelling
F Operant conditioning
G Reciprocal inhibition
H Shaping
I Stimulus generalization

For each of the following vignettes choose one option from the list above which best describes the vignette.

1 A 12-year-old school girl is keen to learn cooking from her mother. As a result, she spends a lot of time in the kitchen with her mother. A week ago, she burnt her fingers while trying to fry chips. Since then, she avoids going near the cooker.

2 A 22-year-old single college student suffers from a phobia of snakes. She attends a therapy session with her clinical psychologist. She is told to sit in a chair and relax while listening to her favourite music and visualising pleasant and relaxing images. She is then shown a picture of a snake.

3 A 10-year-old boy helps his mother by washing the dishes after the family supper. His mother rewards him by giving him an extra helping of the pudding. He quickly learns that every time he helps his mother in any way he gets an extra treat and therefore starts doing that regularly.

[Answers on page 169]

28 Understanding human behaviour on the basis of learning theories

A Chaining
B Classical conditioning
C Cognitive learning
D Covert sensitization
E Learned helplessness
F Modelling
G Negative reinforcement
H Shaping

For each of the following vignettes choose one option from the list above which best describes the vignette.

1   A 39-year-old married woman was a passenger in a car involved in a serious car accident which resulted in the driver's death, about 3 months ago. Now every time she gets into a car, she feels extremely terrified and frightened.

2   A 29-year-old married woman has stopped going out of her house as she feels scared. On two previous occasions when she had gone to the supermarket, she experienced severe dizziness, palpitations and choking with chest pain and had to be taken to the accident and emergency department. She has not experienced such symptoms when she is at home and therefore prefers to stay indoors.

3   A 36-year-old man complains of feeling miserable, unhappy and unmotivated about his life. He believes that nothing he does for his employers or others changes the many adverse stressors in his life.

[Answers on page 170]

29 Identification of ego defence mechanisms

A Acting out
B Denial
C Displacement
D Dissociation
E Distortion
F Externalization
G Reaction formation
H Regression

For each of the following case scenarios choose the option from the list above that could best explain the scenario.

1   An 8-year-old boy previously dry starts wetting his bed. His parents separated recently after the birth of his sister.

2   A 32-year-old married woman becomes verbally and physically aggressive towards her 5-year-old child. Her husband is an alcoholic. He observed this whenever he came back from the pub late in the evening.

3   A 38-year-old woman who was wandering on the street in the middle of the night is brought to the accident and emergency department by her neighbours. She can not give any details of her identity. However, her neighbours said that her husband had died 7 days ago.

[Answers on page 170]

30 Identification of ego defence mechanisms

A Denial
B Dissociation
C Distortion
D Externalization
E Reaction formation
F Regression
G Repression
H Summarization

For each of the following case scenarios, choose one option from the list above that best explains the situation.

1   A 43-year-old man says his wife has gone on holiday for a couple of weeks, so he has to stay at home to look after the dog. He becomes angry whenever his daughter tries to discuss with him the funeral of her mother who died about 3 days ago.

2   A 48-year-old unmarried Asian woman, living with her married brother and his children presents to her general practitioner with multiple physical problems. Her doctor had investigated her thoroughly without any definite organic cause.

3   A 32-year-old woman has developed a habit of handwashing for the last 4 months. She was divorced about 6 months ago. Because of her washing habit, she currently cannot go to work, where she has been employed for the past 10 years.

[Answers on page 170]

31 Identification of ego defence mechanisms that may explain human behaviour

A Denial
B Displacement
C Dissociation
D Idealization
E Identification
F Projection
G Repression
H Sublimation

For each of the following vignettes choose one option from the list above which best describes the vignette.

1   A 35-year-old divorced woman had applied for promotion in her bank. She has worked there for the past 10 years. She was told that her application was unsuccessful, and the job was given to someone younger than her. On her way home, she gets very aggressive towards another driver who overtakes her on the road.

2   The woman in question 1 sees her psychotherapist the next day and describes how her previous day was. The psychotherapist suggests that her reaction while driving could be the result of her anger towards her boss. She said that her boss did not deserve it as he was a nice person and had always been good to her.

3   A 10-year-old boy lives with his parents and 5-year-old sister. His father has to go away frequently on business trips. Whenever he is away, the young boy behaves like his father in looking after his sister.

[Answers on page 170]

32 Identification of ego defence mechanisms

A Displacement
B Idealization
C Intellectualization
D Isolation
E Regression
F Splitting
G Sublimation
H Undoing

For each of the following situations choose the most appropriate option from the list above.

1   A 46-year-old woman was informed by her boss that she would not be promoted, as expected, and the job was given to a younger colleague. While driving home, after finishing work, she was overcome with rage as another car pushed in front of her.

2   The above woman visits her general practitioner and describes her behaviour, which she thought was out of character. The doctor speculated that some of her anger expressed towards other drivers might be linked to her relationship with her boss. However, she replied that this could not be so, as her boss had been like a brother to her, had always been supportive, caring and never critical at any time in the last 4 years.

3   The above woman told her doctor that she had read some undergraduate psychology textbooks. She believed that her sudden and surprising outbursts of anger might be due to her childhood experiences. She then talked at great length on the subject of child-rearing practices in different cultures.

[Answers on page 170]

33 Identification of ego defence mechanisms

A Denial
B Identification
C Isolation
D Projection
E Rationalization
F Reaction formation
G Regression
H Repression

Choose the defence mechanism from the list above which is most likely to be operating in each of the following instances.

1 An 8-year-old boy is brought to his doctor for bed-wetting. He had been successfully toilet trained previously. His mother is expecting another baby soon.

2 A 35-year-old man is traumatized following a serious road traffic accident. He described his experience and the details of the accident in which his 10-year-old son died, without showing any emotion.

3 This phenomenon could explain why so many of us think, 'the good old days' were good.

[Answers on page 170]

Answers

1 Differential diagnosis of genetic disorders

1   B
2   C
3   G

2 Genetics of organic brain disorders

1   H (Rett's syndrome)
2   I (Lesch–Nyhan syndrome)
3   B (Tuberous sclerosis)

3 Differential diagnosis of patients with learning disability

1   H
2   D
3   G

4 Clinicopathological correlations of dementia

1   E, A
2   F, G
3   C, H

5 Behavioural genetics and phenotypes of mental disorders

1   B, E (Rett's syndrome)
2   F, G, I (Prader-Willi syndrome)
3   H, K (Klinefelter syndrome)

6 Mechanism of action of psychoactive chemical substances

1   H
2   A
3   C

7 Mechanism of action of adverse effects of psychotropic drugs

1   G
2   F
3   E

8 Mechanism of action of psychotropic drugs

1   E, H
2   A, C, B
3   F, G

9 Electroencephalographic changes in mental disorders

1   E
2   C
3   B

10 Identification of metabolic/biochemical abnormalities

1   C
2   B
3   G

11 Applications of study designs in clinical research

1   A
2   B
3   G

12 Applications of study designs in clinical research

1   F
2   E
3   F

13 Applications of multivariate analysis in clinical research

1   B
2   A
3   C

14 Applications of multivariate analysis in clinical research

1   H
2   F
3   D, G

15 Identification of bias in research studies

1   F
2   G
3   G

16 Identification of bias in research studies

1   C
2   D
3   A

17 Methods of statistical analysis of research data

1   B
2   H
3   C

18 Methods of statistical analysis of research data

1   F
2   C
3   B

19 Determining appropriate controls in research studies

1   E
2   H, A
3   G

20 Identification of bias in clinical research studies

1   G
2   A
3   H

21 Application of tests of statistical analysis

1	I, C
2	C, J
3	G, F

22 Application of tests of statistical analysis in clinical research

1	C
2	G
3	J

23 Clinical application of learning theories

1	D
2	G
3	C

24 Clinical applications of learning theories

1	B
2	H
3	F

25 Identification of the components of cognitive functions

1	E
2	B
3	I

26 Identification of learning theory underlying human behaviour

1	G
2	F
3	H

27 Understanding human behaviour on the basis of learning theories

1	B
2	G
3	F

28 Understanding human behaviour on the basis of learning theories

1   B
2   G
3   E

29 Identification of ego defence mechanisms

1   H
2   C
3   D

30 Identification of ego defence mechanisms

1   A
2   H
3   E

31 Identification of ego defence mechanisms that may explain human behaviour

1   B
2   D
3   E

32 Identification of ego defence mechanisms

1   A
2   H
3   E

33 Identification of ego defence mechanisms

1   G
2   C
3   H

12 CLINICAL TOPICS: PAPER 1 (ISQs)

Sample questions

General adult psychiatry

1   In acute depersonalization syndrome, there is alteration in tactile perception.

2   In acute depersonalization syndrome, delusional perception is a common experience.

3   In acute depersonalization syndrome, perception of time is significantly altered.

4   In acute depersonalization syndrome, anxiety is usually not experienced.

5   Hyperventilation is a common feature of acute depersonalization syndrome.

6   A persistent difficulty in establishing a sexual relationship is a feature of an obsessional personality.

7   Magical undoing is a recognized feature of an obsessional personality.

8   Fear of dirt is a recognized feature of an obsessional personality.

9   Projection is a recognized feature of an obsessional personality.

10 Excessive preoccupation with cleanliness is a recognized feature of an obsessional personality.

11 Perseveration is a characteristic thought disorder found in patients with schizophrenia.

12 Derailment is a characteristic thought disorder found in patients with schizophrenia.

13 Symbolization is a characteristic thought disorder found in patients with schizophrenia.

14 Neologism is a characteristic thought disorder found in patients with schizophrenia.

15   Thought echo is a characteristic thought disorder found in patients with schizophrenia.

16   Repeated periods of clouded consciousness with intermittent lucid intervals are a recognized feature of Creutzfeldt–Jakob disease.

17   Repeated periods of clouded consciousness with intermittent lucid intervals are a recognized feature of depressive stupor.

18   Repeated periods of clouded consciousness with intermittent lucid intervals are a recognized feature of subdural haematoma.

19   Repeated periods of clouded consciousness with intermittent lucid intervals are a recognized feature of subarachnoid haemorrhage.

20   Repeated periods of clouded consciousness with intermittent lucid intervals are a feature of Wernicke's encephalopathy.

21   Fear of overcrowded places is a characteristic feature of agoraphobia.

22   Fear of going out alone is a recognized feature of agoraphobia.

23   Fear of staying indoors is a characteristic feature of agoraphobia.

24   Fear of traffic is a recognized feature of agoraphobia.

25   Avoidance of public places is a recognized feature of agoraphobia.

26   Ideas of reference is a characteristic feature of Kretschmer's sensitivity reaction.

27   Auditory hallucinations are a characteristic feature of Kretschmer's sensitivity reaction.

28   Shameful inadequacy is a feature of Kretschmer's sensitivity reaction.

29   Rumination about personal achievements is a characteristic feature of Kretschmer's sensitivity reaction.

30   Low threshold for blushing is a feature of Kretschmer's sensitivity reaction.

31   Fear of being unable to control eating is a diagnostic feature of bulimia nervosa.

32   Depressed mood is a diagnostic feature of bulimia nervosa.

33   Insecure sexual relationships are a diagnostic feature of bulimia nervosa.

34   Amenorrhoea is a diagnostic feature of bulimia nervosa.

35   Bulimia nervosa is associated with significant weight loss.

36   Dysmnesic syndrome of recent origin may result from carbon dioxide poisoning.

37   Dysmnesic syndrome of recent origin may result from carbon monoxide poisoning.

38   Dysmnesic syndrome of recent origin may result from ingestion of amphetamines.

39   Dysmnesic syndrome of recent origin may result from nicotinic acid deficiency.

40   Dysmnesic syndrome of recent origin may result from ingestion of lysergic acid diethylamide (LSD).

41   As regards suicide, there is a history of attempted suicide in about 40 per cent of cases.

42   Successful suicide is often preceded by an attempted suicide in the previous three months.

43   As regards suicide, the current trend indicates a shift towards late middle age for the maximum risk of suicide.

44   Individuals with antisocial personality are more likely to commit suicide than the general population.

45   Being married offers some protection against suicide.

46   According to current knowledge, the majority of homosexuals are effeminate.

47   According to current knowledge, the majority of homosexuals are consistently active or passive partners in their relationships.

48   According to current knowledge, the majority of homosexuals have multiple relationships.

49   According to current knowledge, the majority of homosexuals have an identifiable chromosomal or endocrine disorder.

50   According to current knowledge, the majority of homosexuals have an above average sex drive.

51   Persistent facial pain is a variant of migraine.

52   Persistent facial pain is an associated feature of bipolar affective disorder.

53   Persistent facial pain, if it responds to carbamazepine, is likely to be due to trigeminal neuralgia.

54   Persistent facial pain may respond to antidepressant drugs even in the absence of depressed mood.

55   Persistent facial pain may respond to cognitive–behavioural methods.

56   Biological changes seen in patients suffering from mania include increased platelet monoamine levels.

57   Biological changes seen in patients suffering from mania include increased serum cortisol levels.

58   Biological changes seen in patients suffering from mania include reduction in the thyrotrophin releasing hormone response to thyroid releasing factor.

59   Biological changes seen in patients suffering from mania include increased glucose tolerance.

60   Biological changes seen in patients suffering from mania include diffuse abnormalities on electroencephalographic (EEG) recording.

61   The 'main effect' hypothesis suggests that the presence of social support reduces the risk of depression by modifying the impact of adversity.

62   Fregoli's syndrome is an example of delusions of misidentification.

63   Subjective doubles syndrome is an example of delusions of misidentification.

64   Intermetamorphosis syndrome is an example of delusions of misidentification.

65   *Folie a deux* is an example of delusions of misidentification.

66   Short-lived paranoid psychosis with auditory hallucinations is likely to be caused by regular use of barbiturates.

67   Short-lived paranoid psychosis with auditory hallucinations is likely to be caused by regular use of procyclidine.

68   Short-lived paranoid psychosis with auditory hallucinations is likely to be caused by regular use of cannabis.

69   Short-lived paranoid psychosis with auditory hallucinations is likely to be caused by regular use of alcohol.

70   Short-lived paranoid psychosis with auditory hallucinations is likely to be caused by regular use of lysergic acid diethylamide (LSD).

71   According to current knowledge, pharmacological treatments are particularly useful in patients with Gilles de la Tourette's syndrome.

72   According to current knowledge, pharmacological treatments are particularly useful in patients with pica.

73   According to current knowledge, pharmacological treatments are particularly useful in patients with a history of fire setting.

74   According to current knowledge, pharmacological treatments are particularly useful in children with a history of school refusal.

75   According to current knowledge, pharmacological treatments are particularly useful in attention deficit hyperactivity disorder.

76   Homicidal behaviour occurs commonly during the depressed phase of severe bipolar affective disorder.

77   Homicidal behaviour occurs commonly during the manic phase of severe bipolar affective disorder.

78   Homicidal behaviour exhibited by a patient with severe bipolar affective disorder is likely to be directed at the members of his or her family.

79   Homicidal behaviour exhibited by a patient with a severe bipolar affective disorder is invariably followed by suicidal behaviour.

80   Homicidal behaviour exhibited by a patient with a severe bipolar affective disorder represents an alternative to a suicidal attempt.

81   Over-breathing can produce urinary incontinence in a majority of patients.

82   Over-breathing can produce paraesthesia in upper limbs only.

83   Over-breathing can produce profuse salivation in a majority of patients.

84   Over breathing is known to produce carpopedal spasm in both upper extremities.

85   Over-breathing can produce generalized grand mal convulsions in the majority of patients.

86   A background of disruptive family life is found in the majority of people who repeatedly attempt deliberate self-harm.

87   The majority of people who repeatedly attempt deliberate self-harm have a recognized mental disorder according to the International Classification of Diseases (ICD)-10.

88   Long-term unemployment is a characteristic feature of people who repeatedly attempt deliberate self-harm.

89   Residence in a middle-class suburban area is one of the characteristic features of people who repeatedly attempt deliberate self-harm.

90   People with a history of repeated deliberate self-harm are usually of low intelligence.

91   Biological families of patients with schizophrenia show an increase in prevalence of organic brain disorders.

92   Biological families of patients with schizophrenia show an increased prevalence of bipolar affective disorder.

93   Biological families of patients with schizophrenia show an increased prevalence of alcohol-related problems.

94   Biological families of patients with schizophrenia show an increased prevalence of Alzheimer's disease.

95   Biological families of patients with schizophrenia show an increased prevalence of learning disability.

96   Pregnancy in the first trimester is an absolute contraindication to unilateral electroconvulsive therapy.

97   Depressive stupor in a patient with severe learning disability is a contraindication to unilateral electroconvulsive therapy.

98   Acute catatonic schizophrenia is a contraindication to unilateral electroconvulsive therapy.

99   Raised intracranial pressure is an absolute contraindication to unilateral electroconvulsive therapy.

100   A recent cerebrovascular accident is an absolute contraindication to unilateral electroconvulsive therapy.

101   Self-mutilation is a characteristic feature of psychopathic personality disorder.

102   A characteristic feature of psychopathic personality disorder is repeated overdose.

103   Poor impulse control is a characteristic feature of psychopathic personality disorder.

104   A guilt feeling about one's own action is a characteristic feature of psychopathic personality disorder.

105   Homicidal tendency is a characteristic feature of psychopathic personality disorder.

106   Morbid jealousy is commonly associated with alcohol abuse.

107   Morbid jealousy is frequently associated with cocaine abuse.

108   Morbid jealousy is commoner in women than men.

109   Morbid jealousy is often associated with homicide.

110   Morbid jealousy is rarely associated with schizophrenia.

111   In hysterical conversion syndrome, the symptoms reduce conscious anxiety.

112   Hysterical conversion syndrome typically occurs in persons with hysterical personality.

113   In hysterical conversion syndrome, the symptoms are mediated via the autonomic nervous system.

114 In hysterical conversion syndrome, the symptoms are considered symbolic representations of intrapsychic conflicts.

115 In hysterical conversion syndrome, the symptoms disappear as soon as the primary gain is achieved.

116 Hyper-amnesia is a diagnostic feature of major depression.

117 Hyperphagia is a diagnostic feature of major depression.

118 Impaired attention span is a diagnostic feature of major depression.

119 Impaired short-term memory is a diagnostic feature of major depression.

120 Reduced time spent in sleep is a diagnostic feature of major depression.

121 Biochemical changes commonly seen in major depression include an increased thyroid stimulating hormone response to thyrotrophin releasing factor.

122 Biochemical changes commonly seen in major depression include reduced cortisol suppression.

123 Biochemical changes commonly seen in major depression include an increased prolactin level.

124 Biochemical changes commonly seen in major depression include decreased melatonin levels.

125 Biochemical changes commonly seen in major depression include increased adrenocorticotropic hormone levels.

126 Absence seizures are a common cause of drop attacks.

127 Absence seizures are diagnosed by three per second spike and wave activity on an electroencephalogram.

128 Absence seizures usually occur after puberty.

129 Absence seizures respond best to carbamazepine.

130 Absence seizures usually lead to the development of generalized seizures in adult patients.

131 Negativism is most commonly associated with schizophrenia.

132 Automatic obedience is most commonly associated with schizophrenia.

133 Perseveration is most commonly associated with schizophrenia.

134 Blepharospasm is most commonly associated with schizophrenia.

135 Eyelid tremors are most commonly associated with schizophrenia.

136 The International Classification of Diseases (ICD)-10 specifies a minimum duration of 1 month for a diagnosis of depression.

137   The Diagnostic and Statistical Manual of Mental Disorders (DSM)-IV specifies a minimum of 2 months duration for a diagnosis of schizophrenia.

138   The ICD-10 does not specify any time period for the diagnosis of schizophrenia.

139   The ICD-10 is an alphanumeric coding system with a single letter followed by two numbers with a numeric subdivision.

140   DSM-IV is a categorical diagnostic system with operationally defined criteria.

141   Antimuscarinic drugs produce miosis in therapeutic doses.

142   Antimuscarinic drugs are known to produce visual hallucinations.

143   Antimuscarinic drugs are known to increase the probability of tardive dyskinesia.

144   Antimuscarinic drugs reduce the plasma level of neuroleptic drugs.

145   Antimuscarinic drugs should not be prescribed simultaneously with neuroleptic drugs.

146   Tactile hallucinations are a recognized feature in patients with alcoholic polyneuropathy.

147   Tactile hallucinations are a recognized feature in patients with cocaine abuse.

148   Tactile hallucinations are a recognized feature in patients with anorexia nervosa.

149   Tactile hallucinations are a recognized feature in patients with dermatitis artefacta.

150   Tactile hallucinations are a recognized feature of multiple sclerosis.

151   The incidence and prevalence of bipolar affective disorder are higher in males than females.

152   In bipolar affective disorder, the onset of illness is 10–15 years earlier compared with that of unipolar affective disorder.

153   In bipolar affective disorder, there is a familial consistency in treatment responses in both sexes.

154   The incidence of depression in first-degree relatives is higher in bipolar affective disorder than in major depression.

155   The majority of patients with bipolar affective disorder recover fully after a course of lithium carbonate.

156 Tricyclic antidepressant drugs produce cardiac failure due to a negative inotropic effect on the myocardium.

157 Tricyclic antidepressant drugs should not be given to patients with early cataracts.

158 Tricyclic antidepressant drugs are known to produce depersonalization.

159 Tricyclic antidepressant drugs invariably lead to fatal toxicity in serious overdoses.

160 Tricyclic antidepressant drugs should not be combined with lithium carbonate.

161 Erosion of dental enamel is a recognized complication of bulimia nervosa.

162 Parotid gland enlargement is a recognized complication of bulimia nervosa.

163 Epileptic seizures are a recognized complication of bulimia nervosa.

164 Menstrual disturbance is a recognized feature of bulimia nervosa.

165 Peptic ulcer is a recognized complication of bulimia nervosa.

[Answers on page 186]

Old age psychiatry

166 Persecutory delusions occur in about 10 per cent of those over 65 years of age.

167 Persecutory delusions in the elderly usually precede the onset of dementia.

168 Persecutory delusions in the elderly are usually accompanied by Schneider's first rank symptoms.

169 Persecutory delusions in the elderly do not usually respond to antipsychotic drugs.

170 Persecutory delusions in the elderly are usually shared by their partners.

171 As regards self-inflicted harm in elderly people, men are more often involved than women.

172 Self-inflicted harm in elderly people is often precipitated by financial stress.

173 Self-inflicted harm in elderly people carries a lower mortality than in the younger age group.

174 Self-inflicted harm in elderly people is often associated with significant mental disorder.

175   Bereavement is considered to be an important precipitant of self-inflicted harm in elderly people.

176   Hospital admission is essential for a successful treatment of a 75-year-old man with severe depressive illness with psychotic symptoms.

177   A 75-year-old patient with severe depressive illness presents a significantly higher suicidal risk than a 20-year-old severely depressed patient.

178   Electroconvulsive therapy should not be given in a 75-year-old man with severe depressive illness if there is evidence of cognitive impairment.

179   Monoamine oxidase inhibitors are contraindicated in a 75-year-old man with severe depressive illness.

180   A 75-year-old man with severe depressive illness certainly has a shortened life expectancy.

181   Urinary incontinence in the elderly can be reduced by prescribing promazine.

182   Urinary incontinence in the elderly can be reduced by special underclothes (e.g. Kanga pants).

183   Urinary incontinence in the elderly can be reduced by consideration of the design of the ward.

184   Urinary incontinence in the elderly can be reduced by supervision by nursing staff.

185   Urinary incontinence in the elderly can be reduced by toilet training.

186   In Alzheimer's disease, vasodilators are effective in a significant proportion of cases.

187   About 40 per cent of patients with Alzheimer's disease have arteriosclerosis.

188   Alzheimer's disease affects females more than males.

189   Depression is often the first presenting symptom of Alzheimer's disease.

190   In Alzheimer's disease, involuntary movements of hands occur in a majority of patients.

[Answers on page 190]

Addictions

191   Regular consumption of dipipanone may lead to physical dependence.

192   Regular consumption of dihydrocodeine may lead to physical dependence.

193   Regular consumption of orphenadrine may lead to physical dependence.

194   Regular consumption of mirtazapine may lead to physical dependence.

195   Regular consumption of amitriptyline may lead to physical dependence.

196   Lateral nystagmus is a diagnostic feature of Korsakoff's syndrome.

197   Pseudo logia fantastica is a diagnostic feature of Korsakoff's syndrome.

198   A marked suggestibility is a diagnostic feature of Korsakoff's syndrome.

199   Clouding of consciousness is a diagnostic feature of Korsakoff's syndrome.

200   Auditory hallucinations are a diagnostic feature of Korsakoff's syndrome.

[Answers on page 191]

Child and adolescent psychiatry

201   Wide variation in concentration is a recognized feature of children with epilepsy.

202   Nocturnal fits occur in the majority of children with epilepsy.

203   Below average intelligence is a recognized feature of children with epilepsy.

204   *Déjà vu* is a recognized feature of children with epilepsy.

205   School refusal presenting for the first time in a 14-year-old boy is usually associated with antisocial behaviour.

206   School refusal presenting for the first time in a 14-year-old boy is often associated with depression.

207   School refusal presenting for the first time in a 14-year-old boy should be referred to social services rather than a child psychiatrist.

208   School refusal presenting for the first time in a 14-year-old boy would necessitate an immediate change of school.

209   School refusal presenting for the first time in a 14-year-old boy poses a significant risk of development of agoraphobic symptoms in adulthood.

210   Major depression in the mother is an important aetiological factor in failure of bonding.

211   An anankastic personality of the mother is an important aetiological factor in bonding failure.

212   'Participative modelling' is the usual therapeutic approach in bonding failure.

213   Supportive psychotherapy is a useful therapeutic approach in bonding failure.

214   Physical abnormalities in the baby are of little or no significance in the aetiology of bonding failure.

215   Social class differences are found in childhood mental disorders.

216   Social class differences are found in patients who have committed suicide.

217   Social class differences are found in patients with obsessive compulsive disorder.

218   Social class differences are found in patients with anorexia nervosa.

219   Social class differences are found in patients with puerperal psychosis.

220   With reference to language development, children from social class I are more advanced in their speech than those from social class V.

221   With reference to language development, comprehension long precedes the ability to articulate.

[Answers on page 191]

Forensic psychiatry

222   In the UK, 'testamentary capacity' means an ability to give evidence in a court of law.

223   In the UK, the 'Court of Protection' is empowered to give instructions on making a valid will.

224   In the UK, detained psychiatric patients cannot give evidence in the higher law courts.

225   In the UK, 'unfit to plead' results in admission to a special hospital until 'fit to plead' as decided by the Home Secretary.

226   In the UK, 'criminal responsibility' means that children 14 years and over are presumed to be fully responsible.

227   In the UK, approximately 40 per cent of all victims of homicide are children.

228   In the UK, women are responsible for over a third of all homicides in which the offenders are known to suffer from a mental disorder.

229   Sadistic aggressive acts are more likely to occur in response to a need to bolster low self-esteem.

230   A typical profile of an offender with multiple victims includes a tendency to pick strangers as victims.

231   A typical profile of an offender with multiple victims includes the presence of a psychotic disorder.

232   A typical profile of an offender with multiple victims includes socioeconomic groups I and II.

233   In the UK, infanticide is the killing of a child under 12 months of age by a parent.

234   The 'Medea Complex' refers to infanticide in which there is a desire to punish the spouse by killing the children.

235   As regards factitious illness by proxy, the perpetrator frequently has nursing experience.

236   As regards factitious illness by proxy in approximately 50 per cent of cases, there is a history of factitious illness behaviour in the mother.

237   As regards factitious illness by proxy, the perpetrator often appears to be an exemplary mother.

238   Paedophiles, who lack acceptance of the deleterious effects of their sexual behaviour with children, are very resistant to change.

239   Family relationships that do not involve consanguinity generally do not fall within the legal definition of incest in England and Wales.

240   With reference to incest, consent is occasionally a statutory defence to the charge.

241   A father who has an incestuous relationship with his daughter usually suffers from a mental disorder.

242   With reference to shoplifters, mental disorder is a factor in a small number of cases.

243   Recent studies suggest that there is an equal representation of men and women among shoplifters.

244   With reference to arsonists, a sizeable proportion is sexually aroused by the act.

245   A sizeable proportion of arsonists are motivated by revenge, self-protection or anger.

246   The principal motivation for arsonists is the release of despondency and tension by the act of setting a fire.

[Answers on page 192]

Learning disability

247   Microcephaly can occur because of a recessive gene.

248   Microcephaly can occur because of regular smoking during the first two trimesters of pregnancy.

249   Microcephaly can occur because of rubella infection during the third trimester of pregnancy.

250   Microcephaly can occur because of toxaemia of pregnancy.

251   Microcephaly can occur because of exposure to x-ray radiation during pregnancy.

252   In patients with glucose-6-phosphatase deficiency, examination of the eyes provides additional diagnostic support.

253   In patients with Wilson's disease, examination of the eyes provides additional diagnostic support.

254   In patients with Tay–Sachs disease, examination of the eyes provides additional diagnostic support.

255   In a patient with overdose of barbiturate, examination of the eyes provides additional diagnostic support.

256   In colour blindness, examination of the eyes provides additional diagnostic support.

257   Lethargy is a clinical feature of untreated cretinism.

258   A large tongue is a clinical feature of untreated cretinism.

259   Short stature is a clinical feature of untreated cretinism.

260   Normal appearance at birth is a feature of untreated cretinism.

261   Hypotonia is a clinical feature of untreated cretinism.

262   The electroencephalographic changes in Lennox–Gastaut syndrome include diffuse slow spike and wave changes.

263   Temporal variation in the prevalence of severe intellectual impairment does not exist in successive birth cohorts in the same community.

264   Approximately 95 per cent of cases of Down's syndrome are due to disjunction of chromosome 21.

265   Fragile X syndrome is usually associated with a reduction in the size of a repeat sequence near the promoter of a gene called *FMR1*.

266   The gene responsible for fragile X syndrome is on the short arm of the X chromosome at Xq27.

267   In fragile X syndrome multiple repeats of a CGG trinucleotide triplet lead to methylation and silencing of the gene.

[Answers on page 192]

Psychotherapy and psychopathology

268   Supportive psychotherapy is based on the principles of collective unconsciousness.

269   Supportive psychotherapy deals with the impact of chronic physical illness on the patient.

270   The therapist is active and directive in supportive psychotherapy.

271   Supportive psychotherapy is not useful in patients with chronic schizophrenia.

272   Supportive psychotherapy involves cognitive restructuring, reassurance and reinforcement.

273   Supportive psychotherapy is usually concerned with neurotic symptoms.

274   As regards supportive psychotherapy, the emphasis is on problem solving and adaptation in the present.

275   As regards supportive psychotherapy, the patient requires continuous and consistent support of family members.

[Answers on page 193]

Answers

1   False
2   False
3   True
4   False
5   False   Depersonalization syndrome is characterized by the unpleasant state of disturbed perception in which internal parts of body are experienced as changed in various ways. It is associated with mild anxiety, depression and *déjà vu*. Two-thirds of the patients are women.
6   False   It is a feature of psychopathic personality disorder.
7   False   It is a defence mechanism noticed in obsessive compulsive disorder.
8   False   It is a feature of obsessive compulsive disorder.
9   False   It is a defence mechanism not associated with obsessive personality.
10 True
11 False   Persevaration is also observed in other conditions such as dementia and learning disability.
12 True
13 False   Symbolization is one of the mechanisms of dream work.
14 True
15 False
16 False   Creutzfeldt–Jakob disease is a progressive dementia. In depressive stupor, there is no impairment of consciousness.
17 False
18 True
19 False   In subarachnoid haemorrhage, there might be transient impairment of consciousness, which can progress into coma.
20 True
21 True
22 False
23 False
24 True
25 True   Agoraphobia includes a fear of being in places or situations from which escape might be difficult.
26 True
27 False
28 False
29 False
30 False   Kretschmer believed that 'sensitive' people develop suspicious ideas when faced with deeply humiliating experiences. Such ideas can be easily mistaken for persecutory delusion, i.e. sensitive delusion of reference (*Sensitiver Beziehungswahn*).
31 True
32 False
33 False

34 **True**

35 **False** Other diagnostic features of bulimia nervosa include episodes of binge eating and persistent over concern with body shape and weight. Depressed mood is common. Most patients are sexually active.

36 **True**

37 **True**

38 **True**

39 **False** Nicotinic acid deficiency usually causes chronic dysmnesic syndrome.

40 **True**

41 **True** About two-thirds of people who commit suicide have seen a health care worker during the preceding three weeks.

42 **False**

43 **True**

44 **True** People with psychopathic personality disorder commit suicide more often accidentally than with intention.

45 **True**

46 **False**

47 **True**

48 **True**

49 **False** There is no convincing evidence of sex chromosome or neuroendocrine system disorder.

50 **False**

51 **True**

52 **False**

53 **True**

54 **True**

55 **True** Facial pain has many physical causes but it can be relieved by antidepressant drugs, even when there are no depressive symptoms.

56 **True**

57 **True**

58 **True**

59 **False**

60 **False** In mania, glucose tolerance is unaffected and there are no abnormal EEG findings.

61 **False** The 'main effect' hypothesis suggests that the lack of social support directly predisposes to depression.

62 **True**

63 **True**

64 **True**

65 **False**

66 **False**

67 **False**

68 **True**

69 **True**

70 **True**

71 True
72 False
73 False
74 False
75 True   Behavioural modification is useful in pica, fire setting and school refusal.
76 False   Homicidal behaviour is not a common feature in either the depressed or the manic phase.
77 False
78 True
79 False
80 False   It is not an alternative to a suicidal attempt but may be followed by it.
81 False   Over-breathing can lead to increased urinary frequency, paraesthesia in the limbs and dry mouth.
82 False
83 False
84 True
85 False
86 True
87 False
88 True
89 False
90 False   Such people are of average intelligence and come from lower socioeconomic classes. About 10–15 per cent have a detectable mental disorder.
91 False
92 True
93 True
94 False
95 True
96 False   Electroconvulsive therapy is better avoided in the first trimester of pregnancy.
97 False
98 False
99 True
100 True
101 False
102 False
103 True
104 False
105 False   All other features are associated with psychopathic personality but are not considered characteristic of the disorder.
106 False
107 False
108 False

109 **False**

110 **False** Morbid jealousy is associated with alcohol abuse in about 10 per cent of cases. Male to female ratio is 2:1. It is noticed quite often in schizophrenia.

111 **False** They reduce unconscious anxiety.

112 **False** Only about 30 per cent of patients have hysterical personality.

113 **False**

114 **True**

115 **False**

116 **False**

117 **False**

118 **False**

119 **False** All other symptoms except hyper-amnesia occur in depression but are not necessarily diagnostic of depression.

120 **True**

121 **False** Blunted release of thyroid stimulating hormone in response to thyrotrophin releasing factor.

122 **True**

123 **False** Prolactin and adrenocorticotropic hormone levels appear to be unaffected in depression.

124 **True**

125 **False**

126 **False** They are brief disturbances of consciousness without convulsive movements.

127 **True**

128 **False** They usually begin in childhood between 5 and 7 years and cease by puberty.

129 **False**

130 **False**

131 **True**

132 **True**

133 **False** Perseveration is a disorder of speech.

134 **False**

135 **False** Blepharospasm and eyelid tremors may be idiopathic or iatrogenic in origin. They might be seen in patients with schizophrenia.

136 **False** ICD-10 requires a minimum of 2 weeks' duration.

137 **False**

138 **False**

139 **True**

140 **True**

141 **False**

142 **True**

143 **True**

144 **True**

145 **True**

146 **False**

147 True
148 False
149 False
150 False
151 True
152 False   The mean age onset of bipolar affective disorder is slightly higher than unipolar affective disorder.
153 True
154 False
155 False
156 True
157 False   Tricyclic antidepressant drugs can be used quite safely in patients with early cataracts.
158 False
159 False
160 False   They can be used safely with lithium carbonate.
161 True
162 True
163 True
164 True
165 True

Old age psychiatry

166 False   Persecutory delusions are part of late paraphrenia. The prevalence rate is about 0.2–0.3 per cent.
167 False   Paranoid symptoms may precede the onset of dementia and usually respond to antipsychotic medications.
168 True
169 False
170 False
171 True   Unlike deliberate self-harm in young people, men are more likely to be involved in this age group. Mortality ratio is higher than in the younger age group.
172 False
173 False
174 True
175 True
176 True   Electroconvulsive therapy is probably the treatment of choice in depressed elderly patients with psychotic symptoms. They can be successfully treated as outpatients if adequate support is available.
177 True
178 False
179 False
180 True
181 True
182 False

183 True
184 True
185 True
186 False
187 False   Alzheimer's disease is idiopathic in origin and may have genetic basis in some patients. There is no evidence of arteriosclerosis as is the case with multi infarct dementia.
188 True
189 True
190 False

Addictions

191 True
192 True
193 False
194 False
195 False
196 False
197 False
198 False   Such patients are often suggestible.
199 False
200 False

Child and adolescent psychiatry

201 True
202 False
203 False
204 True
205 False   It is an emotional disorder which will require specialist help.
206 True
207 False
208 False   It does not usually require a change of school.
209 True
210 True
211 True
212 True
213 True
214 False   A baby with physical abnormalities may be rejected by the mother.
215 True
216 True
217 False
218 True
219 False
220 True
221 True

Forensic psychiatry

222 **False** 'Testamentary capacity' means the ability to make a valid will.
223 **False** The 'Court of Protection' is empowered to look after the financial affairs of patients.
224 **False**
225 **True**
226 **True**
227 **False** Approximately 15 per cent of the victims are children under 1 year of age. Boys are generally at higher risk than girls.
228 **True** Women are responsible for only 2 per cent of 'normal' homicide in which the conviction was for murder.
229 **True**
230 **True**
231 **False**
232 **False** A typical profile is of a non-psychotic white man of age 20–30 years, socioeconomic class III–IV, who uses a firearm in a dramatic scenario to express resentment and anger at life's frustrations and also his personality difficulties.
233 **False** By the mother.
234 **True**
235 **True** Approximately a third.
236 **False**
237 **True**
238 **True** Unless methods of self-control are developed, re-offending is common.
239 **True**
240 **False**
241 **False** Incest is when a man has sexual intercourse with a female whom he knows to be his daughter, sister, half-sister or mother or when a woman aged 16 permits a man whom she knows to be of such consanguinity to have sexual intercourse with her. Family relationships which do not involve consanguinity, e.g. step-father–daughter, do not fall within the legal definition of incest in England and Wales.
242 **True** Approximately 5 per cent have a substantial mental disorder.
243 **True**
244 **False** A small proportion of the total.
245 **True** They make up at least half of the total referred for psychiatric assessment.
246 **True**

Learning disability

247 **True**
248 **False**
249 **False**
250 **False**

251 **True**

252 **False**

253 **True** In Wilson's disease, golden brown, yellow or green corneal pigmentation is known as Kayser–Fleischer rings.

254 **True** In Tay–Sachs disease, a cheery red macular spot and retinal atrophy lead to blindness.

255 **True**

256 **False**

257 **True**

258 **True**

259 **True**

260 **True**

261 **True**

262 **False** The electroencephalogram shows inter-ictal diffuse slow spike and wave changes. Ictal changes depend on the type of seizure.

263 **False** Temporal variation exists.

264 **False** Non-disjunction.

265 **False** Expansion in gene called *FMR1*.

266 **True**

267 **True**

Psychotherapy and psychopathology

268 **False**

269 **True**

270 **True**

271 **False**

272 **True** Supportive psychotherapy is based on the principle of restoring or strengthening the defences and integrating capacities that have been impaired. It uses the techniques that help the patient feel more secure, accepted, protected, encouraged and safe.

273 **True**

274 **False**

275 **False** Supportive psychotherapy, a type of individual psychotherapy, is used to help a person through the time of crisis. The patient is encouraged to talk about the problems

13 CLINICAL TOPICS: PAPER 2 (ISQs)

Sample questions

General adult psychiatry

1   Depression is a recognized presenting feature of pheaochromocytoma.

2   Depression is a recognized presenting feature of carcinoma of the pancreas.

3   Depression is a recognized presenting feature of hypothyroidism.

4   Depression is a recognized presenting feature of hypoparathyroidism.

5   Depression is a recognized feature of hyperthyroidism.

6   Anorexia is an essential feature of cerebral trypanosomiasis.

7   Insomnia is an essential feature of cerebral trypanosomiasis.

8   Somnolence is an essential feature of cerebral trypanosomiasis.

9   Weight gain is an essential feature of cerebral trypanosomiasis.

10   An elated mood is an essential feature of cerebral trypanosomiasis.

11   Depersonalization syndrome almost always precedes derealization.

12   A primary disturbance of ego functioning is considered to be an aetiological factor of depersonalization syndrome.

13   In depersonalization syndrome, the patient feels that people around him or her have changed.

14   Depressed mood is a characteristic feature of depersonalization syndrome.

15   Depersonalization syndrome usually responds satisfactorily to a course of electroconvulsive therapy.

16   There is a high level of generalized anxiety in the majority of patients with agoraphobic syndrome.

17   Clomipramine is an effective treatment for patients with agoraphobic syndrome.

18   Programmed practice is a treatment of choice for patients with agoraphobic syndrome.

19   There is a higher incidence of sexual problems in female patients with agoraphobic syndrome compared with a controlled population.

20   In agoraphobic syndrome, most patients develop symptoms between the ages of 35 and 40 years.

21   Petit mal epilepsy is usually associated with schizophrenia.

22   Multiple sclerosis is usually associated with schizophrenia.

23   Hyperthyroidism is usually associated with schizophrenia.

24   Parkinson's disease is usually associated with schizophrenia.

25   Diabetes mellitus is usually associated with schizophrenia.

26   Lower socioeconomic class is significantly associated with repetition of deliberate self-harm.

27   Criminal behaviour is significantly associated with repetition of deliberate self-harm.

28   Old age is significantly associated with repetition of deliberate self-harm.

29   Being a male is significantly associated with repetition of deliberate self-harm.

30   Early parental loss is significantly associated with repetition of deliberate self-harm.

31   Fugue states are known to occur in patients suffering from narcolepsy.

32   Fugue states are known to occur in patients suffering from depression.

33   Fugue states are known to occur in patients with severe generalized anxiety disorder.

34   Fugue states are known to occur in patients with psychomotor epilepsy.

35   Fugue states are known to occur in patients experiencing hypoglycaemia.

36   The upper limit for termination of pregnancy in the UK is 24 weeks.

37   In the UK, it is illegal to terminate pregnancy in a girl under the age of 16 years without her consent.

38   In the UK, pregnancy in girls under the age of 16 years of age can only be terminated with the parents' written consent.

39   In the UK, a pregnancy can only be terminated if the patient's General Practitioner agrees.

40   In the UK, two medical certificates are required for termination of pregnancy; one of them must be from a doctor approved under the Mental Health Act 1983.

41   Electroconvulsive therapy is contraindicated in patients with multi-infarct dementia.

42   Electroconvulsive therapy should be used as a treatment of choice in severely depressed elderly patients.

43   Electroconvulsive therapy is not contraindicated in a depressed patient with a recent cerebral vascular accident.

44   Electroconvulsive therapy is the treatment of choice in patients with late paraphrenia.

45   Unilateral electroconvulsive therapy is more effective in the treatment of depersonalization syndrome than bilateral electroconvulsive therapy.

46   Attention span is characteristically impaired in brain damage sustained following a road traffic accident.

47   Attention span is characteristically impaired in patients with hyperkinetic syndrome.

48   Attention span is characteristically impaired in patients with depression.

49   Attention span is characteristically impaired in patients suffering from social phobia.

50   Attention span is characteristically impaired in patients with Pick's disease.

51   Prognosis in patients with obsessive compulsive disorder is better for rituals than ruminations.

52   Prognosis of obsessive compulsive disorder is typically worse in untreated patients than treated patients.

53   Prognosis of obsessive compulsive disorder usually depends on the type of antidepressant drug used.

54   Prognosis of obsessive compulsive disorder can be improved by a combination of selective serotonin reuptake inhibitor drug therapy and behaviour modification techniques.

55   Prognosis of obsessive compulsive disorder is typically worse in patients with a positive family history.

56   A high prevalence of inadequate personality problems is more likely to occur in the biological families of patients with schizophrenia who were brought up by adoptive parents.

57   Epilepsy is more likely to occur in biological families of patients with schizophrenia who were brought up by adoptive parents.

58   A history of first cousin marriages is more likely to be found in the biological families of patients with schizophrenia who were brought up by adoptive parents.

59   Organic brain syndromes are more likely to occur in the biological families of patients with schizophrenia who were brought up by adoptive parents.

60   A high prevalence of alcohol abuse is more likely to occur in the biological families of patients with schizophrenia who were brought up by adoptive parents.

61   Being female is significantly associated with completed suicide in young people with a history of deliberate self-harm.

62   Social class V is significantly associated with completed suicide in young people with a history of deliberate self-harm.

63   Severe personality problems are significantly associated with completed suicide in young people with a history of deliberate self-harm.

64   Broken relationships are significantly associated with completed suicide in young people with a history of deliberate self-harm.

65   Substance misuse is significantly associated with completed suicide in young people with a history of deliberate self-harm.

66   Latent homosexuality may be a primary aetiological factor in sexual difficulties in an otherwise stable marriage.

67   Assortative mating may be a primary aetiological factor in sexual difficulties in an otherwise stable marriage.

68   A fear of pregnancy may be a primary aetiological factor in sexual difficulties in an otherwise stable marriage.

69   Hidden transvestism may be a primary aetiological factor in sexual difficulties in an otherwise stable marriage.

70   Postnatal depression may be a primary aetiological factor in sexual difficulties in an otherwise stable marriage.

71   Auditory hallucinations in clear consciousness are known to occur in atropine poisoning.

72   Auditory hallucinations in clear consciousness are known to occur in amphetamine abuse.

73   Auditory hallucinations in clear consciousness are known to occur in patients who abuse alcohol.

74   Auditory hallucinations in clear consciousness are known to occur in lead poisoning.

75   Auditory hallucinations in clear consciousness are known to occur in patients with Alzheimer's disease.

76   Hypersomnia is a typical feature of liver encephalopathy.

77   Fast electroencephalographic activity is a typical feature of liver encephalopathy.

78   Raised blood ammonia is a typical feature of liver encephalopathy.

79   Impairment of consciousness is a typical feature of liver encephalopathy.

80   Hyperkalaemia is a typical feature of liver encephalopathy.

81   People who cross-dress actively steal clothes from their neighbours' washing lines.

82   Most people who cross-dress do so in the privacy of their own homes.

83   In people who cross-dress, there is usually a confusion of gender identity.

84   Cross-dressing is an act that leads to relief of inner tension.

85   People who cross-dress are usually homosexual in their orientation.

86   Visual hallucinations are a recognized feature of alcoholic hallucinosis.

87   Patients suffering from alcoholic hallucinosis usually present as anxious and restless.

88   Clouding of consciousness is a recognized feature of alcoholic hallucinosis.

89   Many patients who suffer from alcoholic hallucinosis exhibit Schneider's first rank symptoms.

90   Alcoholic hallucinosis may occur at the times of both relative increase and decrease in alcohol intake.

91   Resolution of symptoms when the claim is settled is a typical feature of malingering.

92   In malingering, a family history of the same disorder is common.

93   Frontal headaches are a typical feature of malingering.

94   Fainting attacks are a typical feature of malingering.

95   Severe difficulties with sleep are a typical feature of malingering.

96   Tinnitus is a frequently encountered feature of hyperventilation syndrome.

97   Carpopedal paraesthesias are frequently encountered clinical features of hyperventilation syndrome.

98   Substernal discomfort is a frequently encountered clinical feature of hyperventilation syndrome.

99   Syncope is a frequently encountered clinical feature of hyperventilation syndrome.

100   Nausea and vomiting are frequently encountered clinical features of hyperventilation syndrome.

101   The prevalence of schizophrenia is higher in social classes IV and V than in other social classes.

102   The prevalence of schizophrenia was higher in 1990 than in 1890.

103   The prevalence of schizophrenia is significantly lower in the Republic of Ireland than England and Wales.

104   The prevalence of schizophrenia is higher in monozygotic than dizygotic twins.

105   The prevalence of schizophrenia is significantly higher in India than in the UK.

106   Female gender is a poor prognostic factor for anorexia nervosa.

107   An onset of illness in adolescence is a poor prognostic factor for anorexia nervosa.

108   Binge eating is a poor prognostic factor for anorexia nervosa.

109   Vomiting is a poor prognostic factor for anorexia nervosa.

110   Parental conflict is a poor prognostic factor for anorexia nervosa.

111   Disturbance of recall is a characteristic feature of psychogenic amnesia.

112   Disturbance of retention is a characteristic feature of psychogenic amnesia.

113   Selective loss of memory about oneself is a characteristic feature of psychogenic amnesia.

114   Impairment of short-term memory is a characteristic feature of psychogenic amnesia.

115   Clouding of consciousness is a characteristic feature of psychogenic amnesia.

116   Schneider's first rank symptoms are primary psychological symptoms from which all other symptoms are derived.

117   Schneider's first rank symptoms are known to occur in patients suffering from Alzheimer's disease.

118   Schneider's first rank symptoms are known to occur in patients suffering from bipolar affective disorder.

119   Schneider's first rank symptoms are characteristic features of late onset schizophrenia.

120   Delirious mania is an example of Kraepelin's 'mixed affective states'.

121   Excited depression is an example of Kraepelin's 'mixed affective states'.

122   Depressive stupor is an example of Kraepelin's 'mixed affective states'.

123   Schizoaffective disorder is an example of Kraepelin's 'mixed affective states'.

124   Manic stupor is an example of Kraepelin's 'mixed affective states'.

125   Complex visual hallucinations characteristically occur in multi-infarct dementia.

126   Complex visual hallucinations characteristically occur in Parkinson's disease.

127   Complex visual hallucinations characteristically occur in temporal lobe lesions.

128   Complex visual hallucinations characteristically occur in occipital lobe lesions.

129   Complex visual hallucinations characteristically occur in atypical grief reactions.

130   Papilloedema is a typical feature of communicating hydrocephalus.

131   Neuronal loss in the cerebral cortex is a typical feature of communicating hydrocephalus.

132   Urinary incontinence is a typical feature of communicating hydrocephalus.

133   Bony lesions seen on a skull x-ray are a typical feature of communicating hydrocephalus.

134   Ataxia is a typical feature of communicating hydrocephalus.

135   Latah is characteristically associated with homicidal attacks.

136   Anorexia nervosa is present in all societies across the world.

137   Semen loss syndrome is a type of anxiety disorder found in some cultures.

138   Koro is caused by a viral infection.

139   Amok is found predominantly in Malaysia and South China.

140   Hypochromic anaemia is a characteristic feature of lead poisoning.

141   Pica is a characteristic feature of lead poisoning.

142   Diarrhoea is a characteristic feature of lead poisoning.

143   Wrist drop is a characteristic feature of lead poisoning.

144   An elevated free erythrocyte protoporphyrin is a characteristic feature of lead poisoning.

145   Paroxetine is contraindicated in patients with a history of recent myocardial infarction.

146   Maprotiline is contraindicated in patients with a history of recent myocardial infarction.

147   Mianserin is contraindicated in patients with a history of recent myocardial infarction.

148   Doxepin is contraindicated in patients with a history of recent myocardial infarction.

149   Lofepramine is contraindicated in patients with a history of recent myocardial infarction.

150   Characteristic motor activity is observed in patients with anorexia nervosa.

151   Characteristic motor activity is observed in patients with premenstrual tension syndrome.

152   Characteristic motor activity is observed in patients with Alzheimer's disease.

153   Characteristic motor activity is observed in patients with multiple sclerosis.

154   Characteristic motor activity is observed in patients with Down's syndrome.

[Answers on page 209]

Old age psychiatry

155   Treatment with anticholinergic drugs is an important factor in the aetiology of visual hallucinations in elderly patients.

156   Late paraphrenia is associated with visual hallucinations in elderly patients.

157   Severe visual impairment is an important factor in the aetiology of visual hallucinations in elderly patients.

158   Untreated depression is an important factor in the aetiology of visual hallucinations in elderly patients.

159   Treatment with antihypertensive drugs is an important factor in the aetiology of visual hallucinations in elderly patients.

160   Rapidly fluctuating course is a characteristic feature of multi-infarct dementia.

161   Severe loss of memory in the early stages is a characteristic feature of multi-infarct dementia.

162   There is a preponderance of women among patients with multi-infarct dementia.

163   Multi-infarct dementia is associated with features suggestive of parietal lobe dysfunction.

164   There is reduced activity of choline acetyltransferase in multi-infarct dementia.

165   According to current scientific knowledge, the neurotransmitter changes in Alzheimer's disease include changes to nicotinergic receptors.

166   According to current scientific knowledge, the neurotransmitter changes in Alzheimer's disease include decrease in somatostatin.

167   The Geriatric Depression Scale suggests the possibility of depression if the overall score is 10 or more.

168   The Geriatric Depression Scale is designed to avoid questions concerning somatic symptoms.

169   Factors associated with poorer survival in the patients with Alzheimer's disease include frontal lobe damage.

170   Factors associated with poorer survival in patients with Alzheimer's disease include female gender.

171   Factors associated with poorer prognosis in patients with Alzheimer's disease include prominent behavioural abnormalities.

172   Compared with dementia, sundowning almost always occurs in the patients suffering from delirium.

173   In patients with Alzheimer's disease, disorientation for place is more obvious than that for time.

174   In patients with Alzheimer's disease, disorders of thought content occur in approximately 50 per cent of patients.

175   The CAMCOG is a cognitive subscale of the Cambridge Examination for Mental Disorders of the Elderly.

176   The comprehensive Clifton Assessment Procedure for the Elderly (CAPE) has an information/orientation subscale.

177   According to current scientific knowledge, neurotransmitter changes in Alzheimer's disease include decreased dopamine beta-hydroxylase.

[Answers on page 213]

Addictions

178   Relief drinking is one of the common features of alcohol dependence syndrome.

179   Delirium tremens is one of the common features of alcohol dependence syndrome.

180   Alcoholic hallucinosis is a common feature of alcohol dependence syndrome.

181   Peripheral neuropathy is a common feature of alcohol dependence syndrome.

182   Narrowing of the drinking repertoire is a common feature of alcohol dependence syndrome.

183   Hypertension is a known complication of alcohol dependence syndrome.

184   Parkinson's disease is a known complication of alcohol dependence syndrome.

185   Cerebellar ataxia is a known complication of alcohol dependence syndrome.

186   Oesophageal varices are a known complication of alcohol dependence syndrome.

187   Testicular atrophy is a known complication of alcohol dependence syndrome.

188   The therapeutic action of disulfiram in the treatment of alcohol dependence syndrome depends on the fact that it diminishes the craving for alcohol.

189   The therapeutic action of disulfiram in the treatment of alcohol dependence syndrome depends on the principle of aversion therapy.

190   The therapeutic action of disulfiram in the treatment of alcohol dependence syndrome depends on its immediate metabolite which reverses the sensitivity of receptors for alcohol.

191   The therapeutic action of disulfiram in the treatment of alcohol dependence syndrome depends on the fear of the potentially dangerous interaction with alcohol.

192   The therapeutic action of disulfiram in the treatment of alcohol dependence syndrome depends on its role as a deterrent to impulsive drinking.

193   Excessive alcohol intake is usually associated with cerebellar ataxia.

194   Excessive alcohol intake is usually associated with patients suffering from bipolar affective disorder.

195   Excessive alcohol intake is usually associated with fatty liver.

196   Excessive alcohol intake is usually associated with significant changes in peripheral synaptic transmission.

197   Excessive alcohol intake is usually associated with cardiomyopathy.

[Answers on page 213]

Child and adolescent psychiatry

198   A history of nail biting points to the presence of a psychiatric disorder in an 8-year-old child.

199   A history of thumb sucking points to the presence of a psychiatric disorder in an 8-year-old child.

200   A history of social withdrawal points to the presence of a psychiatric disorder in an 8-year-old child.

201   A history of nocturnal enuresis points to the presence of a psychiatric disorder in an 8-year-old child.

202   Consistent failure to attend school points to the presence of a psychiatric disorder in an 8-year-old child.

203   Being a young mother is usually associated with failure of bonding.

204   An unwanted pregnancy is an aetiological factor of failure of bonding.

205   The baby being nursed in a special care unit is an aetiological factor of failure of bonding.

206   A complicated birth may lead to failure of bonding.

207   Absence of the father of the child in the household may lead to failure of bonding with the mother.

208   Specific reading retardation is present when a child's reading age is two standard deviations below that expected.

209   Specific reading retardation is associated with left–right disorientation.

210   Specific reading retardation is associated with visual defects.

211   With reference to stages of psychosocial development, Freud's oral stage corresponds with Erikson's stage of autonomy.

212   With reference to vision and hearing developmental milestones in a baby, the baby turns its head to sounds at the age of 6 months.

213   With reference to vision and hearing developmental milestones in a baby, the baby will localize sound 18 inches lateral to either ear by the age of 4 months.

214   With reference to developmental milestones, a 3-year-old child can go down the stairs one foot per step.

215   With reference to developmental milestones, a 3-year-old child can dress and undress without assistance.

216   With reference to language development, twins are usually slower to speak than singletons.

217   With reference to a baby's social developmental milestones, it will wave goodbye at 9 months of age.

218   With reference to a baby's social developmental milestones, it drinks from a cup at the age of 1 year.

219   With reference to developmental milestones of speech, a baby makes double-syllable sounds at the age of 6 months.

[Answers on page 214]

Forensic psychiatry

220   A 45-year-old man with previously stable personality is likely to have depression if there is a history of an attempt to kill his wife.

221   A 45-year-old man with previously stable personality is likely to have depression if there is a history of an attempt to kill a passerby.

222   A 45-year-old man with previously stable personality is likely to have depression if there is a history of drunk and disorderly behaviour.

223   A 45-year-old man with previously stable personality is likely to have depression if he is disorientated in time, place and person.

224   A 45-year-old man with previously stable personality is likely to have depression if there is a history of a conviction for indecent exposure.

225   In about three-quarters of murder cases, the victims have known the murderers.

226   In about half of murder cases, homicide suspects kill themselves.

227   The majority of murderers are considered mentally disordered.

228   In British Law, murder is an unlawful killing without malice aforethought.

229   In murder cases, the higher courts have discretion when passing sentence whereas the lower courts have no such privilege.

230   With reference to arsonists, psychotic disorders account for a significant proportion of offenders.

231   With reference to the relation between crime and schizophrenia, those with schizophrenia show a similar rate of offending to the rest of the population.

232   With reference to the relation between crime and schizophrenia, those with schizophrenia are more likely to commit a crime of violence than the rest of the population.

233   Schizophrenic patients with negative symptoms generally commit occasional but often well-planned and serious violence.

234   With reference to offending behaviour, the most commonly assaulted stranger after a public disorder offence is the arresting police officer.

235   With reference to serious sexual offences, there is often a history of persistent uncertainties about sexual orientation.

236   Violence in patients with epilepsy is usually non-goal-directed activity in the ictal phase.

237   Psychotic morbid jealousy shows a poorer outcome after treatment than neurotic morbid jealousy.

238   Patients with Munchausen's syndrome may commit thefts and create disturbances to fund their peregrinations.

239   With reference to offending behaviour, the persistence of normal aspects of personality acts as a break on aggressive behaviour.

240   With reference to offending behaviour, patients with bipolar affective disorder are more likely to be violent to themselves than to others.

[Answers on page 214]

Learning disability

241   A 10-year-old autistic girl is likely to have an attachment to an imaginary friend.

242   A 10-year-old autistic girl may make fleeting gaze contact with the therapist.

243   A 10-year-old autistic girl is likely to have a higher performance score than verbal score in an intelligence test.

244   A 10-year-old autistic girl can only speak by echoing what is said to her.

245   A 10-year-old autistic girl is likely to show manifestations of fragile X syndrome.

246   Hypertelorism is an established cause of severe learning disability.

247   Wilson's disease is an established cause of severe learning disability.

248   Fragile X syndrome is an established cause of severe learning disability.

249   XXY syndrome is associated with severe learning disability.

250   Sanfilippo's syndrome is associated with severe learning disability.

251   XXY chromosomes are a characteristic feature of Klinefelter's syndrome.

252   Gynaecomastia is a characteristic feature of Klinefelter's syndrome.

253   Testicular hypertrophy is a characteristic feature of Klinefelter's syndrome.

254   Severe learning disability is found in the majority of cases of Klinefelter's syndrome.

255   Cataract is a characteristic feature of Klinefelter's syndrome.

256   Above average intelligence is a diagnostic feature of XYY syndrome.

257   Height above average for the general population is a diagnostic feature of XYY syndrome.

258   Large testicles are a diagnostic feature of XYY syndrome.

259   Gynaecomastia is a diagnostic feature of XYY syndrome.

260   Webbing of the neck is a diagnostic feature of XYY syndrome.

261   The Psychiatric Assessment Scale for Adults with Developmental Disability is derived from the Present State Examination.

[Answers on page 215]

Psychotherapy and psychopathology

262   Focus on symptomatic behaviour that occurs in a particular setting, is a characteristic feature of systemic psychotherapy.

263   An interpersonal approach concentrating on dysfunctional relationships in a social group is a characteristic feature of systemic psychotherapy.

264   Systemic psychotherapy involves regular analysis of transference and counter-transference.

265   Systemic psychotherapy is based on principles of systematic desensitization.

266   In systemic psychotherapy, the primary focus is on the individual behaviour in question.

267   In analytic psychotherapy, the therapist must always consider the role of family members in the therapy.

268   In analytic psychotherapy, the therapist must always consider the omissions and errors by the patient.

269   In analytic psychotherapy, the therapist must always consider his or her emotional response to the patient's behaviour.

270   In analytic psychotherapy, the therapist must always consider the sexual content of the patient's behaviour and thoughts.

271   In analytic psychotherapy, the therapist must always consider the implications of the Oedipus complex.

272   In psychoanalytic therapy, resistance is an inevitable phenomenon.

273   In psychoanalytic therapy, resistance is a conscious unwillingness of the patient to continue in the therapy.

274   In psychoanalytic therapy, resistance may be present even if the patient thinks he or she is cooperative.

275   In psychoanalytic therapy, resistance should be dealt with before starting the therapy.

[Answers on page 216]

Answers

1	**True**
2	**True**
3	**True**
4	**True**
5	**True**
6	**True**
7	**True**
8	**True**
9	**False** It is associated with weight loss and apathy.
10	**True**
11	**False**
12	**False**
13	**False**
14	**True**
15	**False** Depersonalization syndrome is characterized by an unpleasant state of feeling unreal and experiencing an unreal quality to perception. On most occasions, it is a secondary condition; and the treatment should be directed to the primary condition.
16	**True** Two peaks of onset: early or middle twenties and mid-thirties.
17	**False**
18	**True**
19	**True**
20	**False**
21	**False**
22	**False**
23	**False**
24	**False**
25	**False** Diabetes mellitus may be associated with depression, anxiety, cognitive impairment, restlessness and irritability.
26	**True**
27	**True**
28	**False**
29	**False** Young females are most likely to repeat acts of deliberate self-harm.
30	**False**
31	**False**
32	**True**
33	**True**
34	**True**
35	**True**
36	**True**
37	**False**
38	**False**
39	**False**

40 False
41 False Contraindications/indications for electroconvulsive therapy are the same whether it is administered unilaterally or bilaterally.
42 True
43 False
44 False
45 False
46 True
47 True
48 True
49 False
50 True
51 False No difference in outcome between rituals and ruminations.
52 True
53 False
54 True
55 False
56 True
57 True
58 False First cousin marriages are more likely to be associated with autosomal recessive disorders.
59 False
60 True
61 False Male sex is a significant factor.
62 True
63 True
64 False
65 True
66 True
67 False
68 True
69 True
70 False
71 False
72 False
73 True
74 False
75 True
76 True
77 False The earliest electroencephalographic change is a slowing of the alpha rhythm and the appearance of 5–7 theta waves per second, which will replace alpha waves as consciousness is progressively impaired. Later, characteristic triphasic waves are seen, suggesting a poor prognosis.
78 True
79 True
80 False

81 **False**

82 **True**

83 **True**

84 **True**

85 **False**

86 **False**   It is characterized by auditory hallucinations, usually voices uttering insult or threats in clear consciousness.

87 **True**

88 **False**

89 **False**

90 **True**

91 **False**   Compensation neurosis is a term used for psychologically determined physical or mental symptoms occurring when there is an unsettled claim for compensation. In some patients, the symptoms may persist for several years after compensation.

92 **False**

93 **True**

94 **True**

95 **False**

96 **False**

97 **True**

98 **True**

99 **True**

100 **False**   The symptoms are due to cerebral vasoconstriction and respiratory acidosis.

101 **True**

102 **False**   There is no evidence that the prevalence was higher or lower in 1990 than in 1890.

103 **False**   High prevalence has been reported in Ireland.

104 **True**

105 **False**   The prevalence is less in India than in the UK as the prognosis is better in the former country.

106 **False**

107 **True**

108 **False**

109 **False**

110 **False**   The only established factor predictive of outcome is the length of illness at presentation. It is also evident that an onset of illness in adolescence and male sex suggests a poor prognosis.

111 **True**

112 **False**

113 **False**

114 **True**

115 **True**   It usually begins abruptly. Some patients report a slight clouding of consciousness during the period immediately preceding the amnesia. The capacity to learn new information is retained in patients.

116 False
117 False
118 True
119 True
120 False
121 True
122 False
123 False
124 True
125 False
126 False
127 True
128 True
129 False
130 False
131 False
132 True
133 False
134 True
135 False   Latah, found in Malaysian women, usually begins after a sudden frightening experience. The patient shows echolalia and echopraxia and is abnormally compliant in other ways.
136 True
137 True
138 False   Koro is a psychogenic disorder, a type of anxiety reaction in which the patient fears that his penis is shrinking and may disappear into his abdomen and that he may die.
139 True
140 True
141 False   Pica is one of the main causes of lead toxicity; the other features include colicky abdominal pain, constipation, headache and irritability. Coma and convulsions occur in severe cases.
142 False
143 True
144 True
145 True
146 True
147 False
148 False   Use with caution in recent myocardial infarction.
149 True
150 True
151 False
152 True
153 False
154 False

Old age psychiatry

155 True
156 True
157 False
158 False
159 False
160 False
161 False
162 False   It is slightly more common in men than women. Emotional and personality changes may appear first followed by impairments of memory and intellect, which fluctuate but not rapidly. There is an association between cognitive impairment and levels of choline acetyltransferase.
163 False
164 False
165 True
166 True   There is also decrease in choline acetyltransferase, acetylcholine, noradrenaline, serotonin, gamma-aminobutyric acid and corticotrophin releasing factor.
167 False   An overall score of 5 or more suggests the possibility of depression.
168 True   Somatic symptoms in older patients might be accounted for by physical disorders.
169 False   Parietal lobe damage is associated with poorer survival rate.
170 False   Male gender.
171 True   For example irritability and wandering.
172 True
173 False   Disorientation for time is more obvious than that for place.
174 False   Disorders of thought content (delusions and paranoid ideation) occur in approximately 15 per cent of the patients.
175 True
176 True
177 True

Addictions

178 True
179 False   Delirium tremens is a withdrawal state.
180 False   Alcoholic hallucinosis is an uncommon complication.
181 False   Peripheral neuropathy is a neurological complication.
182 True
183 False
184 False
185 True
186 True
187 True
188 False   Disulfiram acts by blocking the oxidation of alcohol so that acetaldehyde accumulates, which produces an unpleasant experience.

189 True
190 False
191 True
192 True
193 False
194 False
195 True
196 False
197 True

Child and adolescent psychiatry

198 False
199 False   Nail biting and thumb sucking are considered neurotic traits which have little relevance in psychiatric practice.
200 True
201 True
202 True
203 False
204 True
205 True
206 True
207 False
208 True
209 True
210 True   Also episodic hearing impairments, speech delay, family history of reading difficulties, conduct disorder, large family, etc.
211 False   Freud's oral stage in the first year corresponds with Erikson's trust verses mistrust.
212 False   3 months.
213 False   6 months.
214 False   Two feet per step down stairs and/or one foot per step up stairs.
215 False
216 True
217 False   Usually by 1 year of age.
218 False   By 18 months.
219 True

Forensic psychiatry

220 True
221 False
222 True
223 False
224 True   In depression, aggression is usually directed towards oneself and close family, especially if suicide is contemplated.
225 True

226 **False** Up to 30 per cent of homicide suspects (especially women) kill themselves following murder.

227 **False** About 50 per cent of murderers are mentally disordered and have severe personality disorders.

228 **False**

229 **False**

230 **False** A small proportion of the group.

231 **True**

232 **True** Usually minor in degree.

233 **False** Offences are committed inadvertently or neglectfully.

234 **True**

235 **True** Also a history of institutional rearing, sexual abuse, all in a setting of marked psychological disturbance and low self-esteem.

236 **False** It is usually non-goal-directed activity in the post-ictal phase. Ictal violence is uncommon.

237 **False** Better than neurotic morbid jealousy.

238 **True**

239 **True** Especially in those not habitually prone to using violence to resolve interpersonal difficulties.

240 **True**

Learning disability

241 **True**

242 **True**

243 **True**

244 **False**

245 **False** Fragile X syndrome principally affects males and is the second commonest cause of learning disability after Down's syndrome.

246 **True**

247 **False**

248 **True**

249 **False**

250 **True**

251 **True**

252 **True**

253 **False**

254 **False**

255 **False**

256 **False** Below average intelligence.

257 **True**

258 **False** Testicles are of normal size.

259 **False** A feature of XXY syndrome (Klinefelter's syndrome).

260 **False** A feature of XO (Turner's) syndrome

261 **True**

Psychotherapy and psychopathology

262 True
263 True
264 False
265 False
266 True
267 False   Family members are not involved in such therapy, and nor are conflicts in relation to them dealt with.
268 True
269 True
270 False
271 False
272 True
273 False   Resistance is unconscious interference in therapy which is dealt with as the therapy progresses.
274 True
275 False

14 CLINICAL TOPICS: PAPER 3 (ISQs)

Sample questions

General adult psychiatry

1   The symptoms of acute schizophrenia can be exacerbated in patients taking endorphins.

2   The symptoms of acute schizophrenia can be exacerbated in patients taking L-methionine.

3   The symptoms of acute schizophrenia can be exacerbated in patients taking physostigmine.

4   The symptoms of acute schizophrenia can be exacerbated in patients taking mescaline.

5   The symptoms of acute schizophrenia can be exacerbated in patients taking phencyclidine.

6   Amnesic confabulatory syndrome of longer than several weeks duration is associated with nicotinic acid deficiency.

7   Amnesic confabulatory syndrome of longer than several weeks duration is associated with gastric carcinoma.

8   Amnesic confabulatory syndrome of longer than several weeks duration is associated with carbon monoxide poisoning.

9   Amnesic confabulatory syndrome of longer than a few weeks duration is associated with amphetamine poisoning.

10   Amnesic confabulatory syndrome of longer than a few weeks duration is associated with closed head injury.

11   The rate of suicide is usually lower among Jews and Catholics than among Protestants.

12   The rate of suicide in divorced people is about four times greater than that in married people.

13   Suicide is almost always preceded by an attempted suicide.

14   Suicide rates are usually higher in urban areas than in rural areas.

15 There is a past history of depressive disorder in at least 50 per cent of the victims of suicide.

16 Hypomania can be considered as a probable aetiological factor in a 60-year-old man with a good premorbid personality who exposes himself in a public place for the first time.

17 Erotomania can be considered as a probable aetiological factor in a 60-year-old man with a good premorbid personality who exposes himself in a public place for the first time.

18 Alzheimer's disease can be considered as a probable aetiological factor in a 60-year-old man of good premorbid personality who exposes himself in a public place for the first time.

19 Silent myocardial infarction can be considered as a probable aetiological factor in a 60-year-old man of good premorbid personality who exposes himself in a public place for the first time.

20 Generalized anxiety disorder can be considered as a probable aetiological factor in a 60-year-old man of good premorbid personality who exposes himself in a public place for the first time.

21 A sensitive delusion of reference is a characteristic feature of *sensitiver Beziehungswahn.*

22 An understandable psychological reaction is a characteristic feature of *sensitiver Beziehungswahn.*

23 Ideas of grandeur are a characteristic feature of *sensitiver Beziehungswahn.*

24 Delusional mood is a characteristic feature of *sensitiver Beziehungswahn.*

25 Thought echo is a characteristic feature of *sensitiver Beziehungswahn.*

26 Haloperidol has a sedative effect in therapeutic doses in a majority of patients.

27 Sulpiride has a sedative effect in therapeutic doses in a majority of patients.

28 Risperidone has a sedative effect in therapeutic doses in a majority of patients.

29 Clozapine has a sedative effect in therapeutic doses in a majority of patients.

30 Acute intermittent porphyria is characteristically associated with skin sensitivity to ultraviolet rays.

31 Acute intermittent porphyria is characteristically associated with aspirin compounds.

32   Acute intermittent porphyria is characteristically associated with persecutory delusions.

33   Acute intermittent porphyria is characteristically associated with clouding of consciousness.

34   Acute intermittent porphyria is characteristically associated with red urine.

35   Social class is determined by the Registrar General according to the occupation of the head of the family.

36   A definite relationship exists between social class and suicide.

37   A definite relationship exists between social class and depression.

38   Simple schizophrenia is a subcategory of schizophrenia in the International Classification of Diseases (ICD) -10 classification.

39   Latent schizophrenia is a subcategory of schizophrenia in the ICD-10 classification.

40   Residual schizophrenia is a subcategory of schizophrenia in the ICD-10 classification.

41   Post-schizophrenia depression is a subcategory of schizophrenia in the ICD-10 classification.

42   Schizotypal disorder is a subcategory of schizophrenia in the ICD-10 classification.

43   There is convincing evidence of abnormality of sex chromosomes in homosexual people.

44   As regards homosexuality, there is a significant deficiency of testosterone in the majority of cases.

45   As regards homosexuality, there is a convincing evidence of heredity determining the homosexual behaviour.

46   Most homosexual women engage in a heterosexual relationship at some time in their life.

47   In the majority of patients taking lithium carbonate, it has a stimulating effect in therapeutic doses.

48   In the majority of patients taking fluoxetine, it has a stimulating effect in therapeutic doses.

49   In the majority of patients taking carbamazepine, it has a stimulating effect in therapeutic doses.

50   In the majority of patients taking moclobemide, it has a stimulating effect in therapeutic doses.

51   In the majority of patients taking citalopram, it has a stimulating effect in therapeutic doses.

52   There is a significant risk of suicide associated with obsessive compulsive disorder.

53   There is a significant risk of suicide associated with anorexia nervosa.

54   There is a significant risk of suicide associated with antisocial personality disorder.

55   There is a significant risk of suicide associated with Huntington's disease.

56   There is a significant risk of suicide associated with social phobia.

57   Schizophreniform disorder may be associated more often than by chance with motor neurone disease.

58   Schizophreniform disorder may be associated more often than by chance with hypothyroidism.

59   Schizophreniform disorder may be associated more often than by chance, with diabetes mellitus.

60   Schizophreniform disorder may be associated more often than by chance with Parkinson's disease.

61   Schizophreniform disorder may be associated more often than by chance with multi-infarct dementia.

62   Auditory hallucinations in clear consciousness characteristically occur in lead poisoning.

63   Auditory hallucinations in clear consciousness characteristically occur in Alzheimer's disease.

64   Auditory hallucinations characteristically occur in delirium tremens.

65   Auditory hallucinations in clear consciousness characteristically occur in cocaine abuse.

66   Auditory hallucinations in clear consciousness characteristically occur in mushroom poisoning.

67   Shop-lifting of food is a recognized feature of anorexia nervosa.

68   Increased libido is a recognized feature of anorexia nervosa.

69   Decreased plasma thyroid stimulating hormone (TSH) is a recognized feature of anorexia nervosa.

70   Decreased plasma cortisol is a recognized feature of anorexia nervosa.

71   Inversion of T wave on the electrocardiogram is a recognized feature of anorexia nervosa.

72   Haloperidol is absolutely contraindicated in a patient with a recent history of myocardial infarction.

73   Moclobemide is absolutely contraindicated in a patient with a recent history of myocardial infarction.

74   Clozapine is absolutely contraindicated in a patient with a recent history of myocardial infarction.

75   Fluoxetine is absolutely contraindicated in a patient with a recent history of myocardial infarction.

76   Lithium carbonate is absolutely contraindicated in a patient with a recent history of myocardial infarction.

77   Subjective confusion is a recognized feature of maternity blues.

78   A higher frequency of maternity blues is noted among unmarried mothers.

79   A history of premenstrual tension is associated with maternity blues.

80   A higher frequency of maternity blues is noted among older mothers.

81   Maternity blues are an antecedent of postnatal depression.

82   The majority of patients with fetal rubella syndrome have average intelligence.

83   The majority of patients with neurofibromatosis have average intelligence.

84   The majority of patients with tuberous sclerosis have average intelligence.

85   The majority of patients with athetoid spastic paresis have average intelligence.

86   The majority of patients with spastic paraplegia have average intelligence.

87   Abdominal distension is an essential feature of pseudocyesis.

88   Enlargement of the uterus to a size similar to that at 12 weeks' pregnancy is an essential feature of pseudocyesis.

89   In pseudocyesis, quick resolution occurs on making the correct diagnosis.

90   In pseudocyesis, there is a significant fear of pregnancy.

91   Pigmentation of the breasts is an essential feature of pseudocyesis.

92   Searching behaviour by the bereaved person is an essential feature of a pathological grief reaction.

93   Visual hallucinations are an essential feature of a pathological grief reaction.

94   Auditory hallucinations are an essential feature of a pathological grief reaction.

95   Denial is an essential feature of a pathological grief reaction.

96   Resurrection of the deceased person's last illness is an essential feature of a pathological grief reaction.

97   The term 'haptic hallucinations' is defined as continuous perceptions of vague tingling.

98   The term 'haptic hallucinations' is defined as sensations of temperature change.

99   The term 'haptic hallucinations' is defined as a feeling of movement just below the skin.

100   The term 'haptic hallucinations' refers to an experience of delusional perception.

101   The term 'haptic hallucinations' refers to a phenomenon of tingling and numbness over the abdomen.

102   Paranoid delusions are a diagnostic feature of mania.

103   Disinhibition is a diagnostic feature of mania.

104   Over-spending of money is a diagnostic feature of mania.

105   Over-activity is a diagnostic feature of mania.

106   Transient depressed mood is a diagnostic feature of mania.

107   Mianserin is absolutely contraindicated in a patient with a recent history of myocardial infarction.

108   Imipramine is absolutely contraindicated in a patient with a recent history of myocardial infarction.

109   Maprotiline is absolutely contraindicated in a patient with a recent history of myocardial infarction.

110   Sertindole is absolutely contraindicated in a patient with a recent history of myocardial infarction.

111   Sertraline is absolutely contraindicated in a patient with a recent history of myocardial infarction.

112   The symptoms of acute schizophrenia can be exacerbated by a patient taking L-tryptophan.

113   The symptoms of acute schizophrenia can be exacerbated in a patient taking 5-hydroxytryptamine (5-HT).

114   The symptoms of acute schizophrenia can be exacerbated in a patient taking dopamine.

115   The symptoms of acute schizophrenia can be exacerbated in a patient taking barbiturates.

116   The symptoms of acute schizophrenia can be exacerbated in a patient taking apomorphine.

117   Severe memory impairment is characteristically caused by bilateral hippocampal damage.

118   Lesions in Broca's areas characteristically cause severe memory impairment.

119   Severe memory impairment is characteristically caused by parietal lobe dysfunction.

120   Haemorrhages in mamillary bodies characteristically cause severe memory impairment.

121   Severe memory impairment is characteristically caused by damage to the nucleus accumbens.

122   Blindness is a characteristic feature of methyl alcohol poisoning.

123   Visual hallucinations are a characteristic feature of methyl alcohol poisoning.

124   Vomiting is a characteristic feature of methyl alcohol poisoning.

125   Severe occipital headaches are a characteristic feature of methyl alcohol poisoning.

126   Auditory hallucinations are a characteristic feature of methyl alcohol poisoning.

127   Delusions of guilt are regarded as mood-incongruent in patients suffering from major depression.

128   Hypochondriacal delusions are regarded as mood-incongruent in patients suffering from major depression.

129   The obsessional nature of aggressive thoughts is usually protective against harmful actions.

130   Combined prevalence rates of unipolar and bipolar affective disorders found in the first-degree relatives of bipolar probands are significantly higher than those found in first-degree relatives of unipolar probands.

131   With reference to recovery from depressive disorders, mood-incongruent features have been shown to be predictive of a slower recovery.

132   With reference to recovery from depressive disorders, high neuroticism scores on the Eysenck Personality Inventory are associated with a slower recovery.

133   Predictors of a switch from a depressive episode to a bipolar episode include early age of onset.

134   Predictors of a switch from a depressive episode to a bipolar episode include occurrence in the year after childbirth.

135   With reference to bipolar affective disorder, the first episode is more likely to be triggered by life events than are later episodes.

136   With reference to bipolar affective disorder, flying overnight from east to west is more likely to cause mania than travel in the opposite direction.

137   Factors which predict a good response to lithium prophylaxis in bipolar affective disorder include a family history of the same.

138   Factors which predict a good response to lithium prophylaxis in bipolar affective disorder include the first episode being depression.

139   According to current knowledge, areas of transition between a rural and a more industrialized environment have particularly high morbidity rates for affective disorders.

140   First-degree relatives of unipolar probands have a high risk for bipolar affective disorder, equal to that of the general population.

141   There is an increased risk in relatives of early onset probands of both unipolar and bipolar affective disorders compared with the general population.

142   The 'buffer' theory suggests that lack of social support directly predisposes to depression.

[Answers on page 232]

Old age psychiatry

143   Factors associated with poorer survival in patients with Alzheimer's disease include misidentification phenomena.

144   Hyperorality is a feature of frontotemporal dementia.

145   Preservation of insight is a feature of frontotemporal dementia.

146   Fluent aphasia is a feature of frontotemporal dementia.

147   Spatial disorientation is a feature of frontotemporal dementia.

148   Orientation is more consistently impaired in patients with delirium than with dementia.

149   Depression in all age groups is associated with hypoactivity and upregulation of the hypothalamic–pituitary–adrenal axis.

150   The response of thyroid stimulating hormone (TSH) to thyroid releasing hormone (TRH) is less age dependent than cortisol non-supression.

151   Reminiscence is a recognized psychological treatment for patients with dementia.

152   Validation therapy is a recognized therapy for patients with dementia.

153   Resolution therapy is a recognized psychological treatment for patients suffering from dementia.

154   In elderly patients, the half-life of psychotropic drugs is increased.

155   In elderly patients, there is an increased concentration of water-soluble compounds.

156   Glomerular filtration reduces by up to half by the age of 70 years.

157   Absorption of drugs is significantly altered in elderly patients.

158   Reality orientation is a recognized psychological treatment for patients with dementia.

159   Persecutory delusions are found in approximately 90 per cent of patients with late paraphrenia.

160   Auditory hallucinations are found in approximately 75 per cent of patients with late paraphrenia.

161   Visual hallucinations are detected in up to 60 per cent of patients with late paraphrenia.

162   Schneider's first rank symptoms are frequently seen in patients with late paraphrenia.

163   Degenerative hearing impairment is a recognized risk factor for late paraphrenia.

164   In elderly patients, serum levels of free drugs are higher than in adults.

165   According to current scientific knowledge, the neurotransmitter changes in Alzheimer's disease include increased dopamine.

166   According to current scientific knowledge, the neurotransmitter changes in Alzheimer's disease include increased muscarinic receptors.

[Answers on page 235]

Addictions

167   Alcoholic hallucinosis is characterized by clouding of consciousness.

168   Alcoholic hallucinosis is characterized by visual hallucinations.

169   Alcoholic hallucinosis is characterized by feelings of passivity.

170   Alcoholic hallucinosis is characterized by an upward plantar reflex.

171   Alcoholic hallucinosis is characterized by derogatory auditory hallucinations.

172   Biological markers which may predict vulnerability to developing alcohol-related problems include reduced alpha activity and reduced P300 wave amplitude on electroencephalography.

173   Carbohydrate-deficient transferrin (CDT) is a reliable measure for early recognition of hazardous drinking.

174   Alcohol Use Disorders Test (AUDIT) is least effective at detecting hazardous or harmful drinking.

175   Gamma-glutamyl transpeptidase is raised in at least 90 per cent of heavy drinkers.

176   The rise in cortisol and adrenocorticotrophin (ACTH) following a drink is less among those men with a family history of drinking than in those without.

177   According to current knowledge, dopamine under-activity contributes to the excitability observed in patients with delirium tremens.

178   According to current knowledge, alcohol acts through gamma-aminobutyric acid (GABA) and excitatory amino acid receptors.

[Answers on page 236]

Child and adolescent psychiatry

179   Depressed children often use fantasy to relieve themselves of depression.

180   A majority of untreated depressed children become enuretic in adolescence.

181   In depressed children, social withdrawal is a prominent symptom.

182   Depressed children usually fare less well in school.

183   Persistent stealing from home by 6–10-year-old children is significantly associated with truancy.

184   Persistent stealing from home by 6–10-year-old children is significantly associated with the likelihood of anti-social personality as an adult.

185   Persistent stealing from home by 6–10-year-old children is significantly associated with lack of guilt.

186   Persistent stealing from home by 6–10-year-old children is significantly associated with less pocket money than their friends.

187 Persistent stealing from home by 6–10-year-old children is significantly associated with depressive symptoms.

188 Specific reading retardation is significantly associated with low intelligence.

189 Specific reading retardation is significantly associated with speech delay.

190 Specific reading retardation is significantly associated with spelling difficulties.

191 Specific reading retardation is significantly associated with short-sightedness.

192 Specific reading retardation is significantly associated with school refusal.

193 A large family size is a recognized aetiological factor for increased incidence of delinquency.

194 History of criminality in male siblings is an aetiological factor for increased incidence of delinquency.

195 Low mean intelligent quotient (IQ) is a recognized aetiological factor for increased incidence of delinquency.

196 Parental overprotection is a recognized aetiological factor for increased incidence of delinquency.

197 Low family income is a recognized aetiological factor for increased incidence of delinquency.

198 With reference to motor development milestones in a baby, grasp reflex disappears by the age of 3 months.

199 With reference to motor developmental milestones a baby lets go of objects by the age of 9 months.

[Answers on page 236]

Forensic psychiatry

200 In the UK, a prisoner is not fit to plead if he or she is admitted compulsorily to a psychiatric unit under the Mental Health Act 1983.

201 In the UK, a prisoner is not fit to plead if he or she does not understand the charge (charges) or the significance of their plea.

202 In the UK, a prisoner is not fit to plead if he or she has not reached the age of 14 years.

203 In the UK, a prisoner is not fit to plead if he or she cannot understand the court procedures.

204   In the UK, a prisoner is not fit to plead if he or she experiences active psychotic symptoms.

205   With reference to serious sexual offences, the psychopathology is usually that of unresolved aggressive feelings about significant female figures in the patient's life.

206   With reference to serious sexual offences, there is often a history of cold and affectionless upbringing by unloving parents.

207   Pathological gambling is usually associated with recidivism and other delinquent activities.

208   The absence of *mens rea* forms the basis of the defence of automatism.

209   The legal concept of automatism is the same as the clinical concept of automatic behaviour.

210   Sane automatisms are said to be due to internal causes.

211   Sane automatisms include sleep walking.

212   With reference to dangerousness, previous dangerous behaviour has primacy as a statistical predictor of future violence.

213   According to current knowledge, homicidal offenders are less likely to re-offend than other violent offenders.

214   According to current knowledge, suicide is the second commonest mode of death in prisons.

215   As regards the legal definition of murder in the UK, the offender must be over the age of 10 years.

216   As regards the legal definition of murder in the UK, the offender must not suffer from mental illness.

217   As regards the legal definition of murder in the UK, there is an absence of immediate severe provocation.

218   As regards the legal definition of murder in the UK, there is a proof of unlawful or negligent behaviour.

219   With reference to homicide, the victims are known to the offenders in approximately 50 per cent of homicides.

220   In the UK, males between 10 and 20 years of age account for approximately half of all recorded crimes.

221   Most juvenile offenders attract an International Classification of Diseases (ICD)-10 diagnosis.

222   The age of criminal responsibility is 8 years in Scotland.

223   The commonest of offences in the UK is acquisitive offence.

224 In the UK, age distribution of female offenders is similar to that of males.

[Answers on page 237]

Learning disability

225 As regards severe learning disability, 80 per cent of cases have a known cause.

226 The male-to-female ratio in severe learning disability is 4:1.

227 Prenatal counselling significantly reduces the incidence of severe learning disability.

228 Behaviour modification techniques may improve unhelpful behaviour in the majority of cases of severe learning disability.

229 A characteristic feature of newborn babies with Down's syndrome is generalized hypertonia.

230 A characteristic features of newborn babies with Down's syndrome is a small tongue.

231 A characteristic feature of newborn babies with Down's syndrome is oblique palpebral fissures.

232 A characteristic feature of newborn babies with Down's syndrome is a small and flattened skull.

233 A characteristic feature of newborn babies with Down's syndrome is high cheek bones.

234 Duchenne's muscular dystrophy is X-linked recessive, the abnormal gene being at Xp21.

235 Female carriers of Lesch–Nyhan are mosaic for the condition due to random inactivation of the X chromosome.

236 With reference to fragile X syndrome, multiple copies of a CGG trinucleotide repeat expand down generations particularly when passed through a male meiosis.

237 The somatic phenotype of Prader–Willi syndrome includes hypogonadism and small extremities.

238 The behaviour phenotype of Prader–Willi syndrome includes nonfood related belligerence.

239 Angelman's syndrome includes a small deletion of a differentially imprinted region on the short arm of the paternal chromosome 15.

240 Pica is a clinical feature of Angelman's syndrome.

241 Severe learning disability is a feature of Williams' syndrome.

242   Good verbal ability in contrast to learning disability is a feature of Williams' syndrome.

243   Rett's syndrome occurs only in females.

244   Rett's syndrome is an X-linked recessive condition.

245   The clinical features of West's syndrome include flexor and extensor myoclonic spasms.

[Answers on page 238]

Psychotherapy and psychopathology

246   As regards behaviour therapy for sexual dysfunction, the effect of the presence of both male and female therapists is greater than that of one therapist.

247   As regards behaviour therapy for sexual dysfunction, a ban on sole masturbation is usually necessary.

248   In behaviour therapy, sexual intercourse is banned during the initial phase of treatment of premature ejaculation.

249   Behaviour therapy for sexual dysfunction involves patients keeping a diary of sexual activities.

250   Behaviour therapy does not improve the prognosis of primary erectile impotence.

251   Patients suffering from agoraphobia often show an improvement with intensive short-term psychoanalytic therapy.

252   Patients suffering from dysmorphophobia often show an improvement with intensive short-term psychoanalytic therapy.

253   Patients suffering from nosophobia often show an improvement with intensive short-term psychoanalytic therapy.

254   Patients suffering from irritable bowel syndrome often show an improvement with intensive short-term psychoanalytic therapy.

255   Patients exhibiting transsexualism often show an improvement with intensive short-term psychoanalytic therapy.

256   The first step in family therapy is to identify the context in which symptomatic behaviour occurs.

257   Family therapy aims at helping people to identify their problems in their relationships with others.

258   Family therapy may promote a reorganization of the whole system towards a healthier way of coping.

259   As regards family therapy, the whole family is not always required to be involved in the therapy.

260   Family therapy seeks to stimulate self-help potential of both the patient and key others.

261   The aims of group psychotherapy include an improvement of interpersonal relationships.

262   The aims of group psychotherapy include the conversion of groups into small democratic societies.

263   The aims of group psychotherapy include achievement of significant changes in the people important to the patients.

264   The aims of group psychotherapy include achievement of limited adjustments in a disabling physical illness.

265   The aims of group psychotherapy include the provision of an opportunity to bring about substantial change in psychotic symptoms.

266   Individuals who dominate other people are suitable for group psychotherapy.

267   Individuals who have problems in relating to other people are suitable for group psychotherapy.

268   Individuals who are isolated with their problems are suitable for group psychotherapy.

269   Individuals with a moderate degree of social anxiety are suitable for group psychotherapy.

270   Patients who are unable to establish long-lasting sexual relationships are suitable for group psychotherapy.

271   Crisis intervention is most valuable for well-motivated people with stable premorbid personalities who are facing a major but temporary difficulty.

272   Transference and countertransference are relevant only in dynamic psychotherapy.

273   Cognitive–behavioural therapy is primarily concerned with the pathogenesis of mental disorders.

274   Interpersonal psychotherapy is characterized by its approach as well as its unique techniques.

275   Repeated release of emotion is very important at the beginning of psychological treatments.

[Answers on page 238]

Answers

General adult psychiatry

1   False
2   False
3   False
4   True
5   True   Mescaline and phencyclidine are hallucinogens.
6   True   Untreated nicotinic acid deficiency may lead to a state like Korsakoff's syndrome or slowly progressing dementia.
7   True
8   True
9   False
10 True
11 True
12 False   Suicide rates are lowest among men and are considered higher among the divorced, but certainly not four times.
13 False
14 True
15 True
16 True
17 False
18 True
19 True   Silent myocardial infarction may cause a toxic confusional state, which in turn may lead to antisocial behaviour.
20 False
21 True
22 True
23 False
24 False
25 False   Kretschmer stressed the importance of underlying personality in the development of a delusion. As a sequel to a key experience, delusion develops from sensitive ideas of reference, i.e. *sensitiver Beziehungswahn*.
26 True
27 False
28 False
29 True
30 False   It is characterized by intermittent abdominal pain, peripheral neuropathy, seizures, and psychosis and basal ganglia abnormalities.
31 False
32 False   In acute intermittent porphyria, attacks are precipitated by numerous factors including sulphonamides and barbiturates.
33 False

34   **False**   Freshly voided urine is of normal colour but may turn dark on standing in light and air.
35   **True**
36   **True**   Suicide rates are higher in social classes I and V than in other social classes.
37   **False**
38   **True**
39   **False**
40   **True**
41   **True**
42   **False**   Schizotypal disorder is a separate category under the heading of 'Schizophrenia, schizotypal and delusional disorders'. It is classified as a personality disorder in DSM-IV. It is characterized by eccentric behaviour and abnormalities of thinking and affect which resemble those seen in schizophrenia but without the other characteristic features of schizophrenia.
43   **False**
44   **False**
45   **False**   There is some evidence that homosexual behaviour is determined by heredity but it is not convincing. There is also no convincing evidence of abnormalities in the sex chromosomes or the neuroendocrine system.
46   **True**
47   **False**
48   **True**
49   **False**
50   **True**
51   **True**
52   **False**
53   **True**
54   **True**
55   **True**
56   **False**
57   **False**
58   **True**
59   **False**
60   **True**
61   **True**
62   **True**
63   **True**
64   **True**   In delirium tremens, the hallucinations are associated with clouded consciousness.
65   **True**
66   **True**
67   **True**
68   **False**
69   **True**

70 False   Plasma cortisol is increased and its normal diurnal variation is lost. There is marked reduction in libido at the onset of illness.

71 True

72 True

73 True

74 False

75 False

76 True

77 True

78 False

79 True

80 False

81 False   Maternity blues are more frequent among primipara. The condition is not related to marital status or age of mother. It is certainly not an antecedent of postpartum depression, as it is a self-limiting condition, lasting for a few days.

82 False

83 True

84 False

85 False

86 True

87 True

88 False

89 True

90 True

91 True   Pseudocyesis is the condition of false pregnancy with amenorrhoea, abdominal distension but not necessarily enlargement of uterus, and other changes similar to those of pregnancy.

92 True

93 False

94 False

95 False

96 True   Other features include phobic avoidance of persons, places or things related to the deceased; a total lack of grieving, anger directed towards others, over-idealization of the deceased.

97 True

98 False

99 True

100 False

101 False

102 False

103 True

104 True

105 True

106 True

107 False

108 True
109 True
110 True
111 False
112 False
113 False
114 True
115 False
116 False
117 True
118 False
119 True
120 True
121 False
122 True
123 False
124 True
125 False
126 False   The other features include metabolic acidosis, tachypnoea, confusion, convulsion, and coma.
127 False
128 False
129 True
130 Truc
131 True
132 True
133 True
134 True
135 True
136 False   Travelling from west to east is more likely to cause mania.
137 True
138 False   First episode being mania.
139 True
140 True   0.7 per cent.
141 True
142 False   The 'buffer' theory suggests that the presence of social support reduces the risk of depression by modifying the effect of adversity.

Old age psychiatry

143 False
144 True
145 False   Early loss of insight.
146 False   Non-fluent aphasia.
147 False   Spatial orientation is well preserved.
148 False   It is variably impaired.
149 False   Hyperactivity and dysregulation.

150 True

151 True

152 True Validation therapy focuses on the phenomenology of dementia at an emotional rather than a factual level.

153 True Resolution therapy is a companion to reality orientation. It looks for meaning in the 'here and now' in the confused behaviour of patients with dementia.

154 True Because of increased body fat which acts as a reservoir for those drugs.

155 True Because of reduction in body water.

156 True

157 False Absorption is not grossly affected.

158 True Reality orientation focuses on disorientation and impaired short-term memory.

159 True

160 True

161 True

162 True

163 False Conductive rather than degenerative hearing impairment.

164 True Because of decreased plasma protein/albumin.

165 False Decreased in dopamine.

166 False Decrease in muscarinic presynaptic M_2 receptors.

Addictions

167 False

168 False

169 False

170 False

171 True

172 True

173 True

174 False It is a most effective tool.

175 False It is raised in about 60 per cent of heavy drinkers.

176 True

177 False It is dopamine over-activity.

178 True

Child and adolescent psychiatry

179 False

180 False

181 True

182 True

183 True

184 True

185 True

186 False

187   False   Persistent stealing is a type of conduct disorder which is not significantly associated with depressive symptoms.

188   False   It is associated with impaired writing and spelling and average or above average intelligence.

189   False

190   True

191   False

192   True

193   True

194   True

195   True

196   False

197   True

198   True

199   False   12 months.

Forensic psychiatry

200   False

201   True

202   False   The legal criteria for fitness to plead do not include age and compulsory hospital admission.

203   True

204   False

205   True   Often the mother for whom the victim becomes a surrogate or even a representation of all women.

206   True

207   True

208   True

209   False

210   False   There are external causes.

211   False   This is an insane automatism.

212   True

213   True

214   False   It is the commonest mode of death in prisons.

215   True   A homicide is said to be a murder when the offender is of sound mind and discretion (over age of 10) and had malice aforethought (i.e. intent to cause death or grievous bodily harm).

216   True   This is a mitigating factor for manslaughter.

217   True

218   False

219   False   Approx 75 per cent of British studies.

220   True   The peak age of offending is 14–17 years.

221   False   Only few attract a psychiatric diagnosis.

222   True   In England and Wales, it is 10 years.

223   True   The property offence.

224   True

Learning disability

225 True
226 False
227 True
228 False
229 False
230 False
231 True
232 False
233 False
234 True
235 True   It is also due to a sporadic mutation of *HPRT* general Xq26–27.
236 False   When transmitted through the female.
237 True
238 True
239 False   Patients lack a contribution of maternal chromosome.
240 True
241 False   Mild to moderate learning disability.
242 True
243 True
244 False   X-linked dominant condition.
245 True

Psychotherapy and psychopathology

246 True
247 True   It improves the prognosis of primary erectile impotence but to a
limited extent.
248 True
249 True
250 False
251 False
252 False
253 False
254 False
255 False
256 True
257 True
258 True
259 True
260 True
261 True
262 False
263 False
264 True
265 False

266 False

267 True

268 False   Such people do not benefit from psychotherapy.

269 True

270 True

271 True

272 False   They are relevant in all forms of psychological treatments.

273 False   Its main focus is on the maintenance factors at the time of treatment.

274 False   Its techniques overlap with those of other types of psychotherapy.

275 False   Emotional release can be helpful but repeated release is seldom useful.

15 CLINICAL TOPICS: PAPER 4 (EMIs)

Note: In EMIs each option may be used once, more than once or not at all.

Sample questions

1 Identification of psychiatric defences

A Diminished responsibility
B Insane automatisms
C Negating of *actus rea*
D Negating of *mens rea*
E Pathological intoxication
F Sane automatism
G Testamentary capacity
H Unfit to plead

For each of the following vignettes choose one option from the list above which best describes the vignette.

1   A 35-year-old single unemployed man is charged with the murder of his girlfriend following a night out. He tells his solicitor that he was too drunk at the time of the alleged offence to remember what might have happened.

2   A 52-year-old housewife has a history of uncontrolled partial seizures. She is charged by the police with shoplifting. At the police station, she states that she has no memory of what happened. However, an eye witness saw her stealing something from a store which was confirmed by a close-circuit video recording.

3   A 39-year-old single unemployed man suffers from a chronic enduring and severe psychotic disorder. He is charged with homicide of a member of the public. On examination, he admits to the alleged offence but claims that his voices had told him to kill the 'person'.

[Answers on page 289]

2 Indications of antidepressants for anxiety disorders

A Citalopram
B Clomipramine
C Escitalopram
D Fluoxetine
E Mirtazapine
F Moclobemide
G Paroxetine
H Reboxetine
I Sertraline
J Venlafaxine

For each of the following case scenarios choose the most appropriate option from the list above. Follow the instruction given after each question.

1   A 46-year-old married woman attends the outpatient clinic with a first presentation of previously untreated panic disorder. She has been worried about her daughter's forthcoming wedding. She has noticed that her alcohol intake has increased slightly over the past 6 months. (Choose the three best options.)

2   A 35-year-old married man presents to the outpatient clinic. He has been concerned about his slowness at work since his ritual of checking and rechecking got worse about a year ago. He believes that his performance has dropped below an acceptable level. He feels tormented by ruminations of his day-to-day worries of work. (Choose the three best options.)

3   A 25-year-old single male university graduate presents to the outpatients clinic complaining of blushing, sweating, fine tremors, palpitations whenever he goes out for a drink with his friends. He experiences the same symptoms whenever he goes for a meal in a restaurant. He thinks people are looking at him and consider him to be an inadequate person. However, he does not experience any of these symptoms when he entertains friends at home. (Choose the three best options.)

[Answers on page 289]

3 Identification of distortions of thinking

A Blaming
B Catastrophizing
C Discounting the positive
D Emotional reasoning
E Fantasizing
F Labelling
G Mind reading
H Negative filtering
I Oysterizing

For each of the following situations choose the most appropriate option from the list above.

1   A 36-year-old single female computer programmer attends the clinical psychologist for an assessment of her suitability for cognitive–behavioural therapy. She has been unable to form a stable heterosexual relationship for the past 10 years. During her interview, she repeatedly tells the assessor 'My parents caused all my problems.'

2   A 55-year-old married man, non-executive director of an international company, attends the clinical psychologist for an assessment of his suitability for cognitive–behavioural therapy. During his interview he repeatedly tells his assessor 'My colleagues think I am a failure in my work and my personal life.'

3   A 28-year-old single unemployed male graduate attends the clinical psychologist for an assessment of his suitability for cognitive–behavioural therapy. During the interview he repeatedly tells his assessor 'The university course in physics was easy to pass, so that does not count.'

[Answers on page 289]

4 Clinical applications of cognitive–behavioural therapy

A Cognitive analytical determination of object relations
B Cognitive restructuring of misinterpretation of bodily symptoms
C Dialectical behaviour therapy
D Dropping of safety behaviours, behavioural experiments and video feedbacks
E Establishing hierarchy of fears and engaging in graded exposure
F Exposure and response prevention
G Mindfulness based cognitive therapy
H Schema focused behaviour therapy

For each of the following scenarios choose the most appropriate option from the list above.

1   A 50-year-old married clerical officer presents with a 6-month history of low mood, early morning awakening, lack of energy, reduced interest in life and lack of weight. He seems to be having severe difficulties at work because of repetitive intrusive thoughts that he might cause a serious problem at work by using his computer wrongly. He is concerned that he inputs incorrect data into the computer and spends up to 2 hours daily to check that he has done his work correctly.

2   A 35-year-old single woman presents with a ten-year history of recurrent attacks of shaking, abdominal pain, jelly-like legs, and dizziness when she goes to local pubs and restaurants. At a recent family wedding she had to wash her face every 15 minutes so that others would not notice her sweating and flushed face, which would make them judge her negatively.

3   A 30-year-old single unemployed woman presents with a 5-year history of difficulty in sustaining a job, engaging in a steady relationship and getting angry when they fail. She is looking for a job in a supermarket but fears that she might collapse and die from a heart attack. She had a previous episode when she felt faint while at work. Her father died from a heart attack 2 years ago. On examination, she is found to be medically fit.

[Answers on page 289]

5 Clinical applications of interviewing techniques

A Circular questioning
B Close-ended questions
C Direct questioning
D Facilitation
E Hypothetical questions
F Interpretation
G Paradoxical questions
H Reflection

For each of the following descriptions choose the most appropriate option from the list above.

1 The therapist asks the patient questions such as, 'What does your father say when your mother says this to your sister?'

2 During a family therapy session of a family consisting of a couple, and their daughter and son, the son has been quiet and says very little. On the other hand, the couple and their daughter tend to fill the silence by saying almost anything or having a silly laugh. The therapist asks the couple 'If your son spoke now, what might he say?'

3 During a first family therapy session, the therapist suggests that it is time to take a break. The therapist leaves and the family stay in the room for a few minutes. The therapist then sees his colleague to discuss how the session went so far. The colleague suggests that the family should be carefully advised to continue with what they have been doing so far, i.e. describing their presenting symptoms. All the parties agree to it.

[Answers on page 289]

6 Diagnosis of childhood mental disorders

A Asperger's syndrome
B Attention deficit hyperactivity disorder
C Conduct disorder
D Depressive episode
E Elective mutism
F Gilles de la Tourette's syndrome
G Rett's syndrome
H Transient tic disorder

For each of the following descriptions choose one option from the list above.

1   A 10-year-old boy is brought to the child psychiatrist with a history of poor attention and concentration for the past 2 years. His family and teachers have noticed that he periodically makes strange noises and shows twitches and grimaces.

2   A 12-year-old girl from a stable family presents with a history of repeated hand-washing rituals, episodic over-breathing and unprovoked laughter. She has developed progressive impairment of mobility following early head injury. She is practically housebound.

3   A 16-year-old boy presents with complaints of multiple somatic pains, loss of confidence, lack of interest in his studies and poor concentration. According to his mother, over the last 6 months he has been full of self-reproach and tends to be easily irritated with outbursts of anger.

[Answers on page 289]

7 Clinical management of alcohol-related disorders

A Acamprosate
B Chlordiazepoxide
C Chlormethiazole
D Cognitive–behavioural therapy
E Disulfiram
F Harm reduction programme
G Motivational enhancement therapy
H Simple advice and reassurance
I   12-step programme

For each of the following vignettes choose the most appropriate option from the list above. Follow the instruction given after each question.

1   A 46-year-old married man has a long history of alcohol dependence. He has been almost completely abstinent for 6 months but he finds it increasingly difficult to go without alcohol. He also feels a sense of anxiety in public which makes it further tempting for him to drink. (Choose the three best options.)

2   A 30-year-old, single female company executive drinks two to three glasses of wine every day, especially during weekdays. She believes that she drinks because of her stressful job. She has started to feel ashamed of her daily drinking. She now wishes to cut down to the government recommended 'safe levels' of drinking. (Choose one best option.)

3   A 35-year-old married man was admitted following an attendance in the accident and emergency department after a fall. He informed the nursing staff that he had been drinking heavily for the past 5 years. He was not happy with his life and wants to stop his drinking altogether. The physical investigations reveal severe hepatic and renal impairments. (Choose the three best options.)

[Answers on page 289]

8 Differential diagnosis of anxiety disorders

A Acute stress reaction
B Adjustment disorder
C Bereavement reaction
D Dissociative amnesia
E Mixed anxiety and depression
F Moderate depressive episode
G Post-traumatic stress disorder
H Somatization disorder

For each of the following situations choose one option from the list above which best describes it.

1 A 62-year-old man attends the accident and emergency department with chest pains, palpitations and breathlessness. He was admitted to the medical ward where he soon settles down. He mentioned that he has had trouble with sleep since his flat was burgled 10 days ago. He appeared to have got over the incident and felt reasonably optimistic about the future. However, his main concern is that he does not want to return to his flat.

2 A 55-year-old woman presents to the outpatient clinic with insomnia, recurrent nightmares and depressive symptoms. She was involved in a car crash 5 months back in which she lost her son. She is having phobic avoidance of the site of the crash, which is quite near her house. She is also having problems with concentration and of irritability.

3 A 30-year-old woman presents to the accident and emergency department appearing disoriented and confused. She reported that she had witnessed her husband fall out of the window with their infant son in his arms. When probed further by staff, she becomes irritable and aggressive. She had a seizure 6 hours ago.

[Answers on page 290]

9 Differential diagnosis in neuropathological changes in dementia

A Dementia in Alzheimer's disease
B Dementia in Huntington's disease
C Dementia in Parkinson's disease
D Dementia in Pick's disease
E Frontotemporal dementia
F Multi-infarct dementia
G Subcortical vascular dementia
H Vascular dementia of acute onset

For each of the following descriptions choose the most appropriate option from the list above.

1   There is a marked reduction in the total number of neurones especially in the hippocampus, substantia innominata, locus coeruleus, and temporoparietal and frontal cortices with appearance of neurofibrillary tangles and neuritic plaques.

2   Selective atrophy of the frontal and temporal lobes, but without the occurrence of neuritic plaques and neurofibrillary tangles in excess of those seen in normal ageing.

3   There is a widespread degeneration of the brain, with predominant involvement of the frontal lobe in early stages. This is most marked in the caudate nucleus and basal ganglia.

[Answers on page 290]

10 Diagnosis of uncommon syndromes presenting with learning disability

A Angelman's syndrome
B DiGeorge syndrome
C Lesch–Nyhan syndrome
D Potosi–Shaffer syndrome
E Prader–Willi syndrome
F Smith–Magenis syndrome
G Williams' syndrome
H Wolf–Hirschhorn syndrome

For each of the following choose the best option from the list above.

1   A 7-year-old boy presented to the learning disability outpatient clinic. He has an 'elfin' face, periorbital fullness, star or lacy iris pattern and anteverted nostrils. There is a relative weakness in visuospatial constructive ability with strengths in auditory rote memory and language. Chromosomal studies show microdeletion within the long arm of chromosome 7.

2   A 7-year-old boy presented to the learning disability outpatient clinic. He has a characteristic facial appearance with receding jaw, wide-spaced eyes, a broad bridge of the nose; and mid-face hypoplasia with hypernasal speech. On investigations, he has cardiac abnormalities with absent thymus and hypocalcaemia. Chromosomal studies show that he has microdeletion in chromosome 22.

3   A 7-year-old boy presented to the learning disability outpatient clinic. He has severe learning disability with microcephaly and seizures. The facial appearance is distinctive, with prominent jaws and wide mouth. His gait is ataxic. There is a behavioural phenotype of paroxysmal outbursts of laughter unrelated to prevailing affect or environment and a tendency to tongue thrusting. Chromosomal studies show microdeletion in chromosome 15 of maternal origin.

[Answers on page 290]

11 Managing psychiatric symptoms in patients with dementia

A   An antimuscarinic drug
B   An anxiolytic drug
C   An atypical antipsychotic drug
D   A hypnotic drug
E   A phenothiazine drug
F   A serotonin reuptake inhibitor drug
G   A tricyclic antidepressant drug
H   Environmental optimization
I   Monitoring patient's condition

For each of the following case scenarios, select one option from the list above which will help in the initial management of the patient.

1   A 79-year-old woman on a dormitory ward of an inpatient geriatric medicine unit is found to be acutely confused. She is restless, is pulling on her intravenous line and trying to get out of bed.

2   An 80-year-old man has been admitted to a psychogeriatric ward. Following treatment of a urinary tract infection and additional information from a family member it has became apparent that the mental confusion had been present for 2 years. On two occasions the patient has accused his son of trying to poison him.

3   After discharge from hospital a 75-year-old widow becomes progressively more suspicious over a 3-month period. She telephones her son, making accusations a number of times every day. She refuses to allow her homecare worker into her house. She is also sleeping poorly at night.

[Answers on page 290]

12 Psychiatric diagnosis in the older adults

A Alcohol withdrawal syndrome
B Alzheimer's disease
C Charles Bonnet syndrome
D Cotard's syndrome
E Depression
F Generalized anxiety disorder
G Late-onset schizophrenia
H Obsessive-compulsive disorder
I Reduplicative paramnesia

For each of the following cases, choose one option from the list above which describes it.

1   A 72-year-old previously healthy woman develops a cataract over a period of time. She is functioning quite well. However, over the past few months she describes seeing blue dogs in the corner of her front room.

2   A 70-year-old married executive is admitted to the hospital for a routine surgery. After about 48 hours in hospital and still to have his operation, he becomes acutely confused, anxious and agitated. He experiences prominent and frightening visual illusions.

3   An 89-year-old widower becomes increasingly worried over about 3 months, especially in the mornings. He has lost his confidence and his energy is low. His wife died about 6 months ago.

[Answers on page 290]

13 Physical complications of substance misuse

A Amblyopia
B Hypercalcaemia
C Hyperthermia
D Mallory–Weiss syndrome
E Marchiafava–Bignami syndrome
F Pneumothorax
G Red pustular perinasal rash
H Tricuspid endocarditis
I Wernicke's encephalopathy

For each of the following patients, select one option from the list above which describes the most likely physical complication.

1   A 22-year-old single man presents to the accident and emergency department in an agitated state. He gives a history of multiple poly drug abuse, including injecting, of heroin and cocaine. On examination, he has pyrexia and tachycardia.

2   A 19-year-old previously healthy man is brought to the accident and emergency department in a collapsed state. He had developed acute chest pain after smoking crack cocaine in a local night club.

3   A 17-year-old previously healthy boy was brought to the accident and emergency department by his parents. On examination he has slurred speech, unsteady gait and his breath smells of glue.

[Answers on page 290]

14 Diagnosis of psychiatric disorders with physical symptoms

A Body dysmorphic disorder
B Briquet's syndrome
C Conversion disorder
D Delusional disorder
E Multiple somatoform disorder
F Obsessive-compulsive disorder
G Panic disorder
H Post-traumatic stress disorder
I Schizophrenia
J Somatization disorder

For each of the following cases, select the most appropriate diagnosis from the list of options.

1   A 28-year-old woman presents with a 2-week history of being unable to speak, which began suddenly after witnessing an assault. On examination, she is able to mouth words, but is unable to vocalize. She is noted to cough audibly.

2   The parents of a 28-year-old man are concerned that he has stopped speaking. On examination, he appears fearful, guarded and reluctant to raise his voice above a whisper. When left alone in the examination cubicle, he is observed to shake his head and to make odd movements with his hands.

3   A 42-year-old man takes up to 30 baths every day in an attempt to rid himself of what he describes as an unbearable infestation with lice. His general practitioner says that there is no evidence of such infestation and has found no other evidence of a mental illness.

[Answers on page 291]

15 Management of opiate dependence in a community setting

A Acamprosate calcium
B A viral screen for hepatitis B and C, and human immunodeficiency virus (HIV)
C Buprenorphine tablets
D Intravenous naloxone hydrochloride
E Liver function tests
F Lofexidine tablets
G Methadone mixture (1 mg/mL)
H Methadone tablets (5 mg)
I Naltrexone tablets
J Urine screen for illicit drug, in particular heroin metabolites

For each of the following case scenarios choose the most appropriate initial action from the list above which will help in managing the patient.

1   A 29-year-old man presents to a community drug service with a progressive history of heroin dependence. He is requesting help to come off drugs and abstinence is his goal, although he is fearful of withdrawal symptoms.

2   A 35-year-old man with an established history of heroin dependence of several years duration presents to a community drug service. He is requesting help to come off heroin but does not want to take methadone. He is determined to achieve abstinence at all costs.

3   A 39-year-old man with a history of heroin dependence is on methadone treatment. He attends a drug clinic for his daily dose of methadone. After 60 minutes of receiving 40 mg of methadone he is found slumped in a chair, unarousable, with shallow respiration and pinpoint pupils.

[Answers on page 291]

16 Therapeutic options in the management of depression

A Add carbamazepine
B Add lithium therapy
C Change to a selective serotonin reuptake inhibitor
D Change to a tricyclic antidepressant drug
E Continue the same treatment
F Increase dose of antidepressant drug
G Increase dose of lithium
H Refer for cognitive therapy
I Refer for counselling
J Refer for occupational activity
K Switch to a monoamine oxidase inhibitor
L Use electroconvulsive therapy
M Use a selective serotonin reuptake inhibitor plus a tricyclic antidepressant
drug

For each of the following vignettes choose one option from the list above.

1   A 51-year-old man has recurrent depression. When you saw him 3 weeks ago
     you recommended lithium in addition to amitriptyline he was already taking.
     He continues with low mood and lethargy but his sleep is improving and his
     wife says he is a bit brighter. His lithium level is 0.74 mmol/L.

2   A 31-year-old man with moderate-severe depression for the last 2 years has
     been treated with dosulepin, fluoxetine, venlafaxine and venlafaxine plus
     lithium. He is withdrawn, a little overweight and lethargic. He refuses
     electroconvulsive therapy. He has some counselling and cognitive therapy.

3   A 21-year-old woman is referred by her general practitioner. She has a 6-
     month history of depressive symptoms including low mood, tearfulness,
     lethargy, sleep disturbance and negative thoughts about her. She is struggling
     to look after her young son. She has received a 2-month course of fluoxetine at
     20 mg daily and has been on dosulepin 50 mg for the past 2 weeks.

[Answers on page 291]

17 Diagnosis of substance misuse in the accident and emergency department

A Alcohol
B Amphetamines
C Caffeine
D Cannabis
E Cocaine
F Inhalants
G 'Magic mushrooms'
H Methadone
I Nicotine
J Phencyclidine

For each of the following case scenarios choose the most appropriate options from the list above. Follow the instruction given after each question.

1   A 17-year-old school leaver was brought to the accident and emergency department by his parents. He had gone to an all-night party with his mates. He has a history of abusing illicit drugs for the past 2 years. On physical examination, he has dilated pupils, sweating, labile blood pressure and a mild degree of respiratory depression. (Choose the two best options.)

2   A 19-year-old factory worker was brought to the accident and emergency department by his parents. Since leaving school at 16, he has experimented with a variety of illicit drugs. He had a bad trip last night. On physical examination he has dilated pupils, blurred vision, sweating, tremors and tachycardia. (Choose the two best options.)

3   A 23-year-old single, unemployed man was brought to the accident and emergency department by his family. He had been depressed for several months for no apparent reasons. He started experimenting with illicit drugs 2 months ago. He had exhibited two seizures accompanied by confusion, muscular rigidity, and tachycardia and sweating. (Choose the three best options.)

[Answers on page 291]

18 Clinical application of psychopathology

A Autoscopy
B Capgras' syndrome
C Depersonalization
D Doppelganger
E Erotomania
F *Folie a deux*
G Munchausen's syndrome
H Multiple personality

For each of the following case summaries choose one option from the list above.

1   A 43-year-old unemployed woman went to the police to lodge a complaint against a man. She believes that that man has been coming to her house disguised as her husband to have sex with her. She further informs her doctor that this man looks like her husband and she does not know the actual identity of that man.

2   A 35-year-old unmarried woman, currently an inpatient for 8 hours in the psychiatric unit after a serious suicidal attempt the day before, has no history of alcohol or substance misuse. She is denying her recorded identity and the incident although she explained this act as suicidal at the time.

3   A 32-year-old man with epilepsy presented to his general practitioner with an abnormal head posture. The doctor examined him to exclude any organic pathology. The man said that as he has another neck and head, which other people cannot see, he has to stay in that position.

[Answers on page 291]

19 Movement disorders in patients with schizophrenia

A Automatic obedience
B Catatonia
C Dystonia (acute)
D Mannerism
E Mitgehen
F Parkinsonism
G Tardive dyskinesia
H Waxy flexibility

For each of the following case scenarios, select one option from the list above.

1   A 65-year-old woman with a long history of schizophrenia presents to the outpatient clinic for a review. Her husband says that her mental state has been stable for the past 5 years on an antipsychotic depot injection drug. However, he has noticed that she has been making faces and grimacing at him and other members of the family over the past year.

2   A 35-year-old male patient was seen by a community psychiatric nurse on a home visit. She found him sitting in one corner of the room. His mother informed the nurse that the patient had not eaten for 3 days, nor had he spoken to anyone; he had been passing stools and urine in his clothes during the last day.

3   A 20-year-old man was recently diagnosed as having schizophrenia by his general practitioner. He was prescribed haloperidol in therapeutic doses about 5 days ago. He presents to the accident and emergency department with acute and distressing stiffness and rigidity of his neck since the day before.

[Answers on page 291]

20 Diagnosis of dementia

A Alcohol-related dementia
B Alzheimer's disease
C Communicating hydrocephalus
D Fronto-temporal dementia
E Gerstmann–Strüussler syndrome
F Human immunodeficiency virus (HIV) dementia
G Huntington's disease
H Lewy body dementia
I Multi-infarct dementia
J Parkinson's disease

For each of the case scenarios described below, choose the single most likely diagnosis from the list of options above.

1   A 60-year-old previously healthy woman is referred to the outpatient clinic by her general practitioner. She is accompanied by her husband who reports fluctuating cognitive impairment and visual hallucinations over the past year. At interview she has a mask-like face, slow movements and coarse tremors at rest.

2   A 72-year-old previously healthy man, over the last 2 years has undergone striking changes in his personality and conduct. His speech has progressively deteriorated but his visuospatial ability is relatively preserved.

3   A 80-year-old widower living alone is brought to the accident and emergency department by his neighbours. They have found him wandering at night on several occasions. They have also noticed gradual deterioration in his mental functioning and self-care over the past 3 years. On examination, he could recall his date of birth and address but is disoriented in time, place and person.

[Answers on page 291]

21 Investigations in patients suffering from acute and chronic confusional states

A Arterial blood gas
B Beck Depression Inventory
C Computed tomography (CT)/magnetic resonance imaging (MRI) scan
D Differential blood count
E Full blood count
F Liver function tests
G Mini-Mental State Examination
H Renal function tests
I Serum level of antimanic drug
J Thyroid function tests
K Urine drug screen

For each of the following case scenarios choose the most appropriate options from the list above that will assist in establishing the diagnosis. Follow the instruction given after each question.

1   A 38-year-old woman with a diagnosis of bipolar disorder is admitted after she overdosed on her prescription medication the night before. Her mental state had been stable for several months. She takes her medication regularly and attends her outpatient appointments as required. (Select the three most appropriate investigations.)

2   A 75-year-old man who lives alone is brought in by his daughter as she had noticed that he was becoming increasingly forgetful over the last 2 months. He has difficulty speaking and has a history of hypertension. (Select the two most appropriate investigations.)

3   A 68-year-old woman has been feeling depressed following the death of her husband 7 months ago. She has recently started to become forgetful and has passed urine in her clothes occasionally over the last 2 months. (Select the three most appropriate investigations.)

[Answers on page 292]

22 Diagnosis of motor disorders

A Ambitendency
B Catalepsy
C Cataplexy
D Chorea
E Dystonia
F Echopraxia
G Negativism
H Tics
I Stereotypies

For each of the following choose the most appropriate option from the list above.

1 A 60-year-old man with a long history of schizophrenia lives in a hostel. He had spent 25 years in a mental hospital before he was discharged to the hostel. His antipsychotic drugs were stopped several years ago. He has been noticed to be rocking backwards and forwards, rotating his head and trunk, several times a day.

2 A 45-year-old married woman presents to the accident and emergency department. She gives a history of recurrent falls to the ground often following excitement or laughter.

3 A 30-year-old single woman diagnosed with chronic schizophrenia has been receiving an atypical antipsychotic drug for the past 5 years. Her parents have noticed that when she is on the point of entering a room, she repeatedly walks backwards and forwards across the threshold. When her doctor asked to shake hands, she moved her hand back and forth a few times before completing the gesture.

[Answers on page 292]

23 Management of side effects of psychotropic drugs

A Carbamazepine

B Clonazepam

C Clozapine

D Dantrolene

E Diazepam

F Electroconvulsive therapy

G Madopar (L-dopa and benserazide)

H Procyclidine

I Propranolol

J Tetrabenazine

K L-Tryptophan

For each of the following vignettes choose one option from the list above.

1 A 34-year-old man with learning disability, treated with thioridazine for many years, who develops agitation, muscle rigidity and pyrexia.

2 A 46-year-old solicitor with bipolar affective illness, who has received tricyclic antidepressants and lithium for many years complains of fine tremors of hands for the past 6 months.

3 A 51-year-old woman who has received fluphenazine decanoate for many years because of schizophrenic illness and who exhibits involuntary pursing of the lips.

[Answers on page 292]

24 Pharmacological management of depression

A Chlorpromazine
B Dosulepin
C Fluoxetine
D Imipramine
E Lithium carbonate
F Mianserin
G Mirtazapine
H Moclobemide
I Phenelzine
J Reboxetine
K Venlafaxine

For either of the following case scenarios, select the most appropriate drugs from the list above. Follow the instruction given after each question.

1   A 39-year-old married man is admitted for treatment of mixed anxiety depression. He complains of severe initial insomnia, tiredness and palpitations. When he was treated with amitriptyline he described a 'hang-over' and waking feeling tired and unrefreshed in the morning. (Choose the two best options.)

2   A 42-year-old professional man has been seriously depressed for 6 months. He has not responded to an adequate trial of treatment with amitriptyline and fluoxetine. He had experienced side effects with them. (Choose the two best options.)

3   A 62-year-old woman with a history of recurrent depression attends the outpatients clinic. She has been treated successfully on several occasions with amitriptyline. However, she complained that this caused her problems with sedation, blurred vision and constipation. She had an unsuccessful therapeutic trial with paroxetine. (Choose the two best options.)

[Answers on page 292]

25 Treatment of psychiatric emergencies

A Benztropine
B Bromocriptine
C Dantrolene
D Electroconvulsive therapy
E Folate
F Lorazepam
G Maintaining airway
H Naloxone
I Procyclidine
J Thiamine

For each of the following vignettes choose one or more option from the list above. Follow the instruction after each question.

1 A 30-year-old single man with mild learning disability has been treated with chlorpromazine for several months. He becomes delirious and develops tachycardia, muscular rigidity and pyrexia. (Choose the three best options.)

2 An 18-year-old man who was recently prescribed antipsychotic medication is brought to the accident and emergency department with sustained contraction and twisting of his left hand. (Choose the two best options.)

3 A 44-year-old man who recently underwent emergency appendectomy becomes delirious and experiences visual hallucinations. He has a history of alcohol dependence. (Choose the three best options.)

[Answers on page 292]

26 Differential diagnosis of somatoform and associated disorders

A Conversion disorder
B Diagnosis deferred on axis I of the Diagnostic and Statistical Manual (DSM)-IV
C Factitious disorder
D Hypochondriasis
E Major depressive disorder
F Malingering
G Panic disorder
H Pain disorder
I Somatization disorder

For each of the following vignettes choose one option from the list above which best describes the vignette.

1   A 60-year-old man who was completely asymptomatic until 6 months ago presents to his general practitioner with a preoccupation with his bowel movements. He is convinced that his irregularity represents an occult cancer. Repeated examinations reveal no abnormalities. No occult blood is present in the stools. He had cancelled his prearranged holiday 3 weeks ago as he could not face going abroad.

2   A 45-year-old Iraqi man believes that he is ill because a witch sprinkled 'corpse powder' on his front door and contaminated him is brought to the outpatient clinic. He now has headaches, abdominal pain and no energy. He believes that he will eventually die from this problem. He believes that he saw the witch in the form of a cat at sunset one night.

3   A 35-year-old single woman has been complaining of multiple joint pains, headaches, vomiting, diarrhoea and menstrual irregularities for several years. The physical investigations have proved negative. She believes that she cannot work because of her physical problems.

[Answers on page 292]

27 Clinical application of ICD-10 diagnoses

A Adjustment disorder with prolonged depressive reaction
B Bipolar affective disorder, currently depressed with psychotic symptoms
C Bipolar affective disorder, currently depressed without psychotic symptoms
D Dependent personality disorder
E Depression, currently moderate without somatic syndrome
F Emotionally unstable personality disorder, borderline type
G Histrionic personality disorder
H Cyclothymia
I Recurrent depressive disorder, currently depressed with psychotic symptoms
J Recurrent depressive disorder, currently depressed without psychotic symptoms
K Severe depressive episode with psychotic symptoms

For each of the following vignettes, choose the most appropriate diagnosis from the list above.

1   A 43-year-old woman is brought to the accident and emergency department by ambulance with a history of overdosing on 20 fluoxetine tablets plus analgesics. She has a history of low mood, repeated self-harm, occasionally hearing voices, poor self-esteem and childhood sexual abuse. She is refusing medical treatment for the overdose.

2   A 44-year-old woman presents to her general practitioner with a 3-month history of leukaemia. She describes low mood and poor sleep over the last months but is still able to do her everyday tasks and occasionally enjoys herself.

3   A 45-year-old man presents with depressed mood, anxiety and psychomotor retardation. He feels things are going against him. He is indecisive and has suicidal ideas. He had one similar episode years ago. He is convinced he has a sexually transmitted disease following an affair years ago despite two 'all clear' tests from the genitourinary clinic.

[Answers on page 292]

28 Differential diagnosis of dementing disorders

A Alzheimer's disease
B Communicating hydrocephalus
C Frontal lobe dementia
D Gerstmann-Strüussler syndrome
E Human immunodeficiency virus (HIV) dementia
F Huntington's disease
G Multi-infarct dementia
H Lewy body dementia
I Parkinson's disease
J Pick's disease

For each case scenario described below choose the single most appropriate diagnosis from the above list of options.

1   A 64-year-old man with a history of subarachnoid haemorrhage presents with an 8-month history of progressive ataxia, and urinary incontinence. Lately, he has also become forgetful. At the interview, he looked apathetic with psychomotor slowing.

2   A 58-year-old man with no previous psychiatric history and stable personality was caught shoplifting. At the interview, he underestimates the seriousness of his action and dismisses it with inappropriate jocularity. He is well oriented in time, place and person with minimal memory impairment.

3   A 62-year-old man who lives alone, with a history of hypertension and transient ischaemic attacks presents with self-neglect and poor compliance with his medication. He appears to have difficulties in managing his daily activities. At the interview he is aphasic and irritable, denying all his problems.

[Answers on page 293]

29 Diagnosis of somatoform and associated disorders

A Conversion disorder
B Factitious disorder
C Hypochondriasis
D Major depressive disorder
E Malingering
F Pain disorder
G Panic disorder
H Somatization disorder

For each of the following vignettes choose one option from the list above which best describes the vignette.

1 A 31-year-old divorced woman who was previously healthy presents with sudden loss of sensation and flaccid paralysis of her entire left arm. Her two young children were taken into care a few days ago.

2 A 33-year-old married previously healthy woman presents to the accident and emergency department with complaints of episodic chest tightness and breathing difficulties that started recently. She was previously healthy. The physical investigations are negative.

3 A 32-year-old single man is referred from the gastroenterology department for complaints of unexplained diarrhoea. He has been a frequent attendee at the general practice over the last 5 years following his divorce, with complaints relating to headaches, chest pains, difficulty in breathing and problems with passing urine and stools. Previously he was a manager in a bank and but has been off sick from work for over 2 years.

[Answers on page 293]

30 Differential diagnosis of anxiety disorders

A Acute stress reaction
B Agoraphobia with panic disorder
C Agoraphobia without panic disorder
D Dissociative amnesia
E Dissociative fugue
F Mixed anxiety and depression
G Post-traumatic stress disorder
H Panic disorder
I Trance and possession disorder

For each of the following scenarios choose the best option from the list above.

1   A 24-year-old single Asian woman is brought to the accident and emergency
    department by her parents. They inform you that she has been behaving
    strangely since the break up of her engagement 2 days ago. She has been
    speaking in a strange tone of voice and making strange noises, has been
    wearing very dramatic make-up and was going around in circles in her room,
    saying that she is a goddess and will punish all those who have wronged her.

2   A 23-year-old single woman is brought to the accident and emergency
    department by her parents. They inform you that she had gone missing from
    home 3 days ago after the break up of her engagement. They had reported her
    missing to the police. She was brought back home this morning by the police
    who found her wandering about in the neighbouring town. She was unable to
    give them any details about how she got there or where she had been for the
    last 3 days.

3   A 26-year-old single woman is brought to the accident and emergency
    department by her parents. They inform you that she has been acting strangely
    for a couple of hours. She had been assaulted and robbed at knifepoint by a
    masked man earlier in the evening and since then she has been extremely
    agitated, has been crying and appearing quite confused. She is also very
    anxious and appeared very frightened even at the appearance of her father
    from work this evening.

[Answers on page 293]

31 Differential diagnosis of disorders of perception

A *Echo de la pensée*
B Extracampine hallucinations
C Formication
D Functional hallucinations
E Hypnagogic hallucinations
F Lilliputian hallucinations
G Micropsia
H Pareidolia
I Reflex hallucinations

For each of the following descriptions choose the best option from the list above.

1 A 27-year-old single man tells you that Satan talks to him whenever he starts the tap and hears the running water. He finds that very distressing and therefore has refused to wash or drink from running water for the last 3 months.

2 A 27-year-old single man informs you that whenever he sees Tony Blair on the television, he gets a sharp pain in his abdomen which has convinced him that Tony Blair is controlling him through the television and interfering with his bodily functions.

3 A 45-year-old man who has had an emergency appendectomy informs you that he can see tiny pink elephants dancing on the window-sill. He has a history of alcohol dependence.

[Answers on page 293]

32 Differential diagnosis of delusional disorders

A Capgras' syndrome
B Cotard's syndrome
C De Clerambault's syndrome
D Delusional intuition
E Delusional perception
F Ekbom's syndrome
G *Folie imposée*
H Retrospective delusion

For each of the following descriptions choose the best option from the list above.

1 A 28-year-old man has been arrested by the police after he stabbed a passerby with a knife. On questioning, he said that while he was standing at a crossing, the light turned red as soon as the victim approached the crossing, he then knew that the man was evil and God would like to have him punished and therefore he stabbed him.

2 A 28-year old man who had been diagnosed as having schizophrenia 5 years ago informed his doctor that when he was 16 he underwent an operation for appendectomy. He now knows that at that time, a chip was inserted in his abdomen which allowed the government to monitor his every move and keep an eye on him.

3 A 55-year-old woman has been living with her schizophrenic husband for the past 25 years. She told her doctor that she was inclined to agree with her husband that their neighbours had planted devices in their house to overhear their conversations. She also believed that her neighbours were part of an elaborate terrorist organization that soon planned to bomb London's West End. She then said that her husband was no longer mentally ill.

[Answers on page 293]

33 Differential diagnosis of personality disorders

A Anankastic personality disorder
B Anxious (avoidant) personality disorder
C Dependent personality disorder
D Dissocial personality disorder
E Emotionally unstable personality disorder
F Enduring personality change after catastrophic experience
G Histrionic personality disorder
H Paranoid personality disorder
I Schizoid personality disorder

For each of the following descriptions choose the best option from the list above.

1   A 25-year-old woman was admitted following an overdose of 10 paracetamol
     tablets. She was wearing a lot of make-up and a party outfit. She said that she
     took the overdose when she saw her boyfriend talking to an attractive woman,
     but now regrets it as he had apologized to her. She said that she had recently
     had breast augmentation surgery. She was smiling inappropriately while talking
     about the overdose.

2   A 25-year-old woman is referred as she has been feeling low and has some
     sleep problems. During the interview she tells the doctor that she did not really
     want to see a psychiatrist as her partner of 9 years did not approve it. He is 10
     years older than her and has always taken care of her. She does not want to
     offend him. He takes care of all the finances and gives her money only for the
     grocery shopping but she knows that he is better at managing their lives.

3   A 25-year-old married woman is seen together with her husband because of
     her increasing difficulty in intimacy with her husband over the last 2 years. This
     started after she was taken hostage by two men, who repeatedly sexually
     assaulted her for 5 days. She has also stopped socializing and has become very
     suspicious of everyone. She always feels anxious and 'on the edge'. She had
     been diagnosed as having post-traumatic stress disorder after the incident and
     has been treated for the same.

[Answers on page 293]

34 Differential diagnosis of behavioural and emotional disorders occurring in childhood

A Disinhibited attachment disorder of childhood
B Elective mutism
C Hyperkinetic disorder
D Reactive attachment disorder of childhood
E Separation anxiety disorder of childhood
F Social anxiety disorder of childhood
G Socialized conduct disorder
H Unsocialized conduct disorder

For each of the following descriptions choose the best option from the list above.

1 A single mother brings her 12-year-old son to the outpatient clinic. She says that he has become increasingly unruly over the past year. He has been quite rude to her, answers back all the time and often lies to her. He has often played truant from school and has now been suspended for setting off the fire alarm. She has noticed that he has been hanging out with some older boys who are known to be troublemakers.

2 A 5-year-old girl is brought to the outpatient clinic by her parents who have recently adopted her from a care home. She was at the care home from the age of 1 year. She seems to be excessively friendly with strangers and often tries to be the centre of attention. One of the workers in the home mentioned to them that as a toddler she was very clingy and often cried when the care worker left in the evenings.

3 The mother of an 8-year-old girl brings her to the outpatient clinic as she is having increasing difficulty in getting her daughter to go to school. The daughter had always been anxious about going to school and that has · gradually increased to such an extent that she has not attended school for a month. She is constantly worried that something bad will happen to her mother if she is away from her.

[Answers on page 293]

35 Differential diagnosis of mental disorders in the elderly

A Bereavement
B Charles Bonnet syndrome
C Cotard's syndrome
D Delirium tremens
E Dementia
F Late-onset schizophrenia
G Moderate depressive episode
H Mixed anxiety and depression
I Recurrent depressive disorder

For each of the following descriptions choose the best option from the list above.

1   A 72-year-old woman presents to the elderly services feeling quite low in mood. She mentioned that her husband passed away quite suddenly due to a heart attack 6 months ago. Since then she has been having difficulty sleeping, she cries quite often and does not feel like eating or going out. She sometimes feels that she has felt her husband's presence, especially during the night when she is falling asleep. She has a past history of depression.

2   A 62-year-old executive 48 hours after admission undergoes major surgery. Soon after surgery he becomes disorientated and agitated and has visual hallucinations.

3   A 75-year-old woman developed cataract few months ago. She has been physically well. She presents with increased paranoia and mentions that she has been seeing strange people in her bathroom.

[Answers on page 294]

36 Use of laboratory investigations in confirming a diagnosis

A Arterial blood gases
B Cholesterol levels
C Creatinine kinase
D Fasting blood sugar
E Full blood count
F Gamma-glutamyl transferase
G Liver function tests
H Serum prolactin levels
I Thyroid function

For each of the following descriptions choose the most appropriate investigation from the list above.

1   A 20-year-old man on antipsychotics is admitted with fever and rigidity and labile blood pressure.

2   A 25-year-old single woman on antipsychotics presents with delayed periods and galactorrhoea.

3   A 45-year-old male patient on acamprosate with a past history of alcohol dependence presents with tremulousness, anxiety and disturbed sleep. He tells you he has been abstinent for the past 2 years.

[Answers on page 294]

37 Differential diagnosis of somatoform disorders

A Depressive disorder
B Factitious disorder
C Hypochondriasis
D Neurasthenia
E Panic disorder
F Persistent delusional disorder
G Somatization disorder
H Undifferentiated somatoform disorder

For each of the following case scenarios choose the option from the list above that best describes the option.

1   A 39-year-old single woman was admitted to a medical ward recently complaining of headaches, chest pains, heartburns, dyspepsia, diarrhoea, difficulty with micturition and intermittent heavy and prolonged menstrual bleeding. She has been investigated extensively over a number of years for a variety of symptoms with lumbar puncture, magnetic resonance imaging (MRI) scan, nerve conduction studies, echocardiograms, endoscopy, barium meal, and dilatation and curettage, but without conclusive results.

2   A 45-year-old married Nigerian man attends the outpatient clinic with complaints of weakness, blurred vision and headaches. He believes his symptoms are due to nocturnal ejaculation which started a year ago. The physical examination is unremarkable. He is not willing to accept any other explanation.

3   A 30-year-old single, unemployed woman has repeated admissions to hospitals with complaints of haematuria and painful sexual intercourse. Several investigations including repeated cystoscopy have been consistently normal. The urology team are at a loss to explain her symptoms.

[Answers on page 294]

38 Differential diagnosis of psychosomatic symptoms/syndromes

A Body dysmorphic disorder
B Conversion disorder
C Hypochondriasis
D Illness behaviour
E Sick role
F Somatization disorder
G Type A ◄— behaviour
H Type B ◄— behaviour
I Undifferentiated somatoform disorder

For each of the following vignettes choose one option from the list above which best describes the vignette.

1   A 45-year-old married middle-ranking hospital manager presents to the outpatient clinic with headaches, abdominal pain, palpitations, sleep disturbance and feeling anxious for the past 6 weeks. His general practitioner has signed him off sick 4 weeks ago. He tells his psychiatrist that his employers have transferred some of his main responsibilities to one of his junior colleagues 8 weeks ago. He is compliant with his treatment but is not getting better, although he is keen to do so and return to his work at an earliest possible opportunity.

2   A 54-year-old married doctor has been suffering from mild angina attacks intermittently for the past 2 years. His colleagues see him as a highly ambitious, dynamic go-getter.

3   A 42-year-old married woman attends the outpatient clinic with complaints of excessive tiredness, loss of appetite, nausea, vomiting, diarrhoea and difficulty with micturition for the past 8 months. She has consulted various specialists who have told her that there was nothing seriously wrong with her. She believes that she is unable to fulfil her role as a housewife. She denies any history of drug or alcohol abuse.

[Answers on page 294]

39 Differential diagnosis of memory disorders

A Anterograde amnesia
B Cryptomnesia
C Global amnesia
D Post-traumatic amnesia
E Pseudo logia fantastica
F Psychogenic amnesia
G Retrograde amnesia
H Transient global amnesia

For each of the following situations choose one option from the list above.

1   A 62-year-old man makes a witty remark in a conversation with his friends. He does not recall that he had heard it on television the night before.

2   A 30-year-old man presents himself to the accident and emergency department. He appeared mildly confused but is able to tell his address but not his name or date of birth. He is alert and is orientated to time and place.

3   A 33-year-old married woman is diagnosed with histrionic personality disorder and seems to be in serious trouble with the law. At the interview, it transpires that her statements were often grandiose and extreme but untruthful.

[Answers on page 294]

40 Differential diagnosis of personality disorders

A Anankastic personality disorder
B Avoidant personality disorder
C Borderline personality disorder
D Dissocial (antisocial) personality disorder
E Histrionic personality disorder
F Narcissistic personality disorder
G Schizoid personality disorder
H Schizotypal personality disorder

For each of the following vignettes choose one option from the list above which best describes the vignette.

1   A 29-year-old single unemployed man attends the accident and emergency department repeatedly following fights with strangers in the local pub. He is adamant that he is never to be blamed for his behaviour. He claimed that each of the four times he was sent to prison for violent behaviour was the result of miscarriage of justice. He reveals that he has fathered three children with different partners. He has been with a new partner for 3 months and does not see his children much.

2   A 21-year-old single man is taken to his general practitioner by his mother who is worried about him, although he does not see any problem in himself. He works on an assembly line. For several years he has not engaged in normal social activities, preferring his own company. He does not have any friends, and spends most of his time watching television in his bedroom.

3   A 32-year-old single female company executive attends the outpatient clinic. She is smartly dressed and wearing a lot of make-up. She appeared to take a great pride in her appearance. She has a labile affect. Her clinical history seemed to have several inaccuracies although she laughed these off when they are pointed out to her.

[Answers on page 294]

41 Differential diagnosis of eating disorders

A Anorexia nervosa
B Atypical bulimia nervosa
C Bulimia nervosa
D Depression
E Hyperthyroidism
F Hypothyroidism
G Inflammatory bowel syndrome
H Somatization disorder
I Tuberculosis

For each of the following vignettes choose the best option from the list above.

1   A 17-year-old female is seen in the outpatient clinic. She is accompanied by her mother. She has been referred by her general practitioner who informs you that the patient's body mass index (BMI) is 16.5. She is refusing to follow the prescribed diet as she is very worried about putting on weight. She wishes to pursue a career in modelling and therefore is very careful about her looks and is unable to understand why others are so concerned about her weight.

2   A 32-year-old single woman is seen in the outpatient clinic. She gives a long history of mood swings and self-harming behaviour by cutting. She informs that her boyfriend recently left her and since then her long-term eating problem has worsened. Although she binges on food quite often, she induces vomiting to avoid getting fat.

3   A 36-year-old woman presents with a history of intermittent episodes of mood change and anxiety has been complaining of despair, poor concentration, erratic sleep pattern, excessive eating and a significant weight gain. According to her all her problems started following the discovery of her husband's infidelity 6 months ago. At the interview, she feels inadequate as a wife and is ashamed of her weight.

[Answers on page 294]

42 Drug treatment of substance misuse

A Acamprosate
B Buprenorphine
C Bupropion
D Disulfiram
E Lofexidine
F Methadone
G Naloxone
H Naltrexone

For each of the following clinical scenarios of patients presenting with substance misuse disorders choose one first line of treatment.

1   A 25-year-old single, male factory worker presents to the substance misuse clinic. He tells the staff that he has a 'habit' and injects heroin regularly. He is fed up with his lifestyle. He has been in trouble with the law and misses work frequently. He wants to stop taking heroin but is worried about withdrawal symptoms.

2   A 31-year-old man with a history of heroin abuse was released from prison 3 days ago. While in the prison for 6 months, he did not have heroin. His girlfriend who is on methadone brought him to the accident and emergency department. On arrival, he was unconscious and had pinpoint pupils. She tells the staff he took only a small amount of her heroin a few hours ago.

3   A 29-year-old single unemployed woman has just completed an inpatient detoxification programme. She has a history of recurrent heroin abuse over the past 5 years. She requests medication to help with relapse prevention.

[Answers on page 295]

43 Drug treatment of withdrawal states

A Antimanic drugs
B Antimuscarinic drugs
C Antipsychotic drugs
D Anxiolytics
E Barbiturates
F Hypnotics
G Monoamine oxidase inhibitors
H Non-opioid analgesics
I Serotonin selective reuptake inhibitors
J Vitamin B complex

For each of the following vignettes choose options from the list above. Follow the instruction given after each question.

1   A 38-year-old male company executive was admitted to the hospital 4 days ago. He had sustained a compound fracture of the left tibia after a fall. He was making an uneventful recovery following an operation, however, he is noticed to have periods of intermittent confusion, tremors, vivid hallucinations and illusions. (Choose the three best options.)

2   A 26-year-old single man is brought to the accident and emergency department by his parents as he has become excitable, unpredictable and aggressive over the past 3 days. He is noticed to be depressed and yawning. He complained of nausea, vomiting and diarrhoea. On examination, he had raised temperature and rhinorrhea. (Choose the two best options.)

3   A 32-year-old single woman is brought to the accident and emergency department by her partner as she has been excitable, angry and sleeping for long hours over the past 4 days. She complains of tiredness, vivid unpleasant dreams and increased appetite for the past 3–4 days. She admits heavy use of unspecified stimulants for a few years. (Choose the two best options.)

[Answers on page 295]

44 Mechanisms of adverse drug interactions

A Alpha-2 blockade
B Blockade of mesolimbic D_2 receptors
C Blockade of striatal D_2 receptors
D Induction of liver enzymes
E Inhibition of liver enzymes
F Muscarinic blockade
G Stimulation of histaminic receptors
H Stimulation of 5-hydroxytryptamine 1A (5-HT_{1A}) receptors

For each of the following clinical situations, select one option from the list above.

1   A 36-year-old depressed woman is under treatment with fluoxetine. She supplements this with St John's wort (*Hypericum perforatum*). Despite taking her oral contraceptive pills regularly, she finds herself pregnant.

2   A 45-year-old depressed man is being treated with fluoxetine but responds only partially after 10 weeks. Fluoxetine is augmented with lithium carbonate. The next day, he develops mild confusion, sweating, tachycardia and tremulousness.

3   A 62-year-old man with atrial fibrillation being treated with warfarin is prescribed fluvoxamine for depressive illness. He develops extensive bruising over his body.

[Answers on page 295]

45 Differential diagnosis of somatoform disorders

A Briquet's syndrome
B Concussion
C Conversion disorder
D Dissociative amnesia
E Fugue
F Korsakoff's syndrome
G Hypochondriasis
H Psychogenic pain disorder
I Retrograde amnesia

For each of the following clinical situations, select the best option(s) from the list above. Follow the instruction given after each question.

1   A 35-year-old previously healthy Gulf War soldier had returned home from his duties a few months ago. He has now been asked to rejoin his colleagues. He suddenly finds his right hand paralysed. (Choose one best option.)

2   A 26-year-old man attends the accident and emergency department complaining of being hit on the head while crossing the road, which he claimed occurred 3 days earlier, in a town some 60 miles away. On further enquiry, he could not recall his name or address or how he arrived at the hospital. However, he is aware of the day and date. (Choose the two best options.)

3   A 35-year-old married woman consults her general practitioner complaining of abdominal pain, nausea and bloating. Her physical examination is normal, as is a subsequent range of investigations. The medical notes indicate that over the past 5 years, she had attended repeatedly with a wide range of complaints, including pain at various sites, menstrual disturbances and double vision. She has consulted several specialists, who have not been able to identify physical causes sufficient to explain her symptoms. (Choose the two best options.)

[Answers on page 295]

46 Pharmacological management of psychotic disorders

A Antimanic drugs
B Antimuscarinic drugs
C Antipsychotic depot injection
D Anxiolytics
E Atypical antipsychotic drugs
F β-blockers
G Hypnotics
H Phenothiazines
I Serotonin reuptake inhibitors
J Tricyclic antidepressant drugs

For each of the following clinical situations, select the best option(s) from the list above. Follow the instruction given after each question.

1   A 46-year-old man has been hospitalized five times in the past year, for relapse of symptoms. With each hospitalization, he quickly recompensates with monitored medication and the ward milieu. (Choose one best option.)

2   A 35-year-old single woman has chronic paranoid delusions and persistent derogatory auditory hallucinations. She shows a lack of spontaneity and creativity. She is unemployed and finds it difficult to motivate herself to do anything outside her flat. (Choose the three best options.)

3   A 26-year-old single woman with a previous psychotic episode has been drug free for 1 year. Recently, she started experiencing acute and florid auditory hallucinations of the demon telling her to kill her neighbours because they had poisoned her water supply. (Choose the two best options.)

[Answers on page 295]

47 Pharmacological treatment of depression

A Amitriptyline
B Citalopram
C Desipramine
D Dosulepin
E Fluoxetine
F Lofepramine
G Mirtazapine
H Phenelzine
I Reboxetine
J Sertraline
K Duloxetine
L Venlafaxine

For each of the following vignettes choose the most appropriate options from the list above. Follow the instruction given after each question.

1   A 45-year-old company executive with mixed anxiety depression for about a year complains of marked insomnia. He was initially prescribed imipramine. This was discontinued as he complained of 'hang over and feeling unrefreshed in the mornings'. (Choose the two best options.)

2   A 40-year-old married professional woman has been severely depressed for 10 months. She has not responded to an adequate therapeutic trial of paroxetine and mianserin. Her medication compliance is good. (Choose the two best options.)

3   A 65-year-old widow has a history of multiple episodes of depression. She has been treated successfully on several occasions with imipramine. However, she complains that this caused blurred vision and constipation. (Choose the three best options.)

[Answers on page 295]

48 Risk factors for common mental disorders

A Childhood sexual abuse
B Female gender
C Hypertension
D Impaired hearing
E Insulin resistant syndrome
F Living alone
G Male gender
H Severe osteoarthritis
I Stroke

For each of the following case histories choose options from the list above. Follow the instruction given after each question.

1   A 72-year-old man is referred from the geriatric ward. He has been showing increasing problems with his memory following a fall recently. He now has weakness of his left arm and difficulty speaking. (Choose the three best options.)

2   A 67-year-old female is referred by her general practitioner. Her daughter has been increasingly worried about her following the death of her father 10 months ago. She has been getting paranoid about her neighbours, and believes that they had installed cameras in her house. She says she can also hear her neighbours talking about her through the walls and they often say negative things about her. (Choose the three best options.)

3   A 25-year-old woman often presents to the accident and emergency department with repeated attempts of self-harm by overdosing or cutting herself. She has a history of low mood, low self-esteem and anorexia nervosa. She also often drinks excessively and uses illicit substances. (Choose the two best options.)

[Answers on page 295]

49 Investigations in patients with acute and chronic confusional states

A Arterial blood gases
B Blood culture
C Blood glucose
D Brain computed tomography (CT)/magnetic resonance imaging (MRI) scan
E Full blood count
F Liver function tests
G Lumber puncture
H Midstream urine culture
I Renal function tests
J Skull X-ray
K Thyroid function tests
L Urinary drug screen

For each of the following clinical scenarios, choose the most appropriate options that will assist in establishing the diagnosis. Follow the instruction given after each question.

1   A 51-year-old woman was admitted to hospital with social withdrawal, loss of interest, psychomotor retardation and poor food intake. She suddenly develops chest pains and breathlessness. On examination, she is tachypnoeic and has a pleural rub. (Choose the three best options.)

2   A 32-year-old man with a history of intravenous drug abuse develops night sweats, fatigue and arthralgia. On examination, he has widespread petechiae and splenomegaly. (Choose the two best options.)

3   A 20-year-old Algerian student was brought to the accident and emergency department by his friends. He had been exhibiting erratic and strange behaviour for the past 6 hours. He had been working hard for his forthcoming examination. He looks frightened and talks about police tapping his phone for suspected terrorism. (Choose one best option.)

[Answers on page 296]

Answers

1 Identification of psychiatric defences

1   D
2   B
3   A

2 Indications of antidepressants for anxiety disorder

1   A, C, G
2   B, D, I
3   B, F, G

3 Identification of distortions of thinking

1   A
2   G
3   C

4 Clinical applications of cognitive–behavioural therapy

1   F
2   D
3   E

5 Clinical applications of interviewing techniques

1   A
2   E
3   D

6 Diagnosis of childhood mental disorders

1   F
2   G
3   D

7 Clinical management of alcohol-related disorders

1   A, D, E
2   H
3   B, C, E

8 Differential diagnosis of anxiety disorders

1   B
2   G
3   A

9 Differential diagnosis in neuropathological changes in dementia

1   A
2   D
3   B

10 Diagnosis of uncommon syndromes presenting with learning disability

1   G
2   B
3   A

11 Managing psychiatric symptoms in patients with dementia

1   H
2   I
3   C

12 Psychiatric diagnosis in the older adults

1   C
2   A
3   E

13 Physical complications of substance misuse

1   H
2   F
3   G

14 Diagnosis of psychiatric disorders with physical symptoms

1   C
2   I
3   D

15 Management of opiate dependence in a community setting

1   J
2   F
3   D

16 Therapeutic options in the management of depression

1   E
2   K
3   F

17 Diagnosis of substance misuse in the accident and emergency department

1   B, G
2   B, G
3   B, E, J

18 Clinical application of psychopathology

1   B
2   H
3   A

19 Movement disorders in patients with schizophrenia

1   G
2   B
3   C

20 Diagnosis of dementia

1   H
2   D
3   B

21 Investigations in patients suffering from acute and chronic confusional states

1   H, J, I
2   C, G
3   B, C, G

22 Diagnosis of motor disorders

1   I
2   C
3   A

23 Pharmacological treatment of side effects of psychotropic drugs

1   D
2   I
3   J

24 Pharmacological management of depression

1   G, K
2   G, K
3   E, K

25 Treatment of psychiatric emergencies

1   D, F, I (Neuroleptic malignant syndrome)
2   A, I (Dystonic reaction)
3   C, D, G (Delirium tremens)

26 Differential diagnosis of somatoform and associated disorders

1   E
2   B
3   I

27 Clinical application of ICD-10 diagnoses

1   F
2   A
3   I

28 Differential diagnosis of dementing disorders

1 B
2 C
3 G

29 Diagnosis of somatoform and associated disorders

1 A
2 G
3 H

30 Differential diagnosis of anxiety disorders

1 I
2 E
3 A

31 Differential diagnosis of disorders of perception

1 D
2 I
3 F

32 Differential diagnosis of delusional disorders

1 E
2 H
3 G

33 Differential diagnosis of personality disorders

1 G
2 C
3 F

34 Differential diagnosis of behavioural and emotional disorders occurring in childhood

1 G
2 A
3 E

35 Differential diagnosis of mental disorders in the elderly

1   A
2   D
3   B

36 Use of laboratory investigations in confirming a diagnosis

1   C
2   H
3   F

37 Differential diagnosis of somatoform disorders

1   G
2   F
3   B

38 Differential diagnosis of psychosomatic symptoms/syndromes

1   E
2   G
3   I

39 Differential diagnosis of memory disorders

1   B
2   F
3   E

40 Differential diagnosis of personality disorders

1   D
2   G
3   E

41 Differential diagnosis of eating disorders

1   A
2   C
3   D

42 Drug treatment of substance misuse

1   F
2   G
3   H

43 Drug treatment of withdrawal states

1   C, D, J
2   C, H
3   D, I

44 Mechanisms of adverse drug interactions

1   D
2   H
3   E

45 Differential diagnosis of somatoform disorders

1   C
2   D, E
3   A, G

46 Pharmacological management of psychotic disorders

1   C
2   C, E, H
3   E, H

47 Pharmacological treatment of depression

1   G, F
2   A, L
3   C, F, L

48 Risk factors for common mental disorders

1   C, G, I (Vascular dementia)
2   B, D, F (Late-onset schizophrenia)
3   A, B (Borderline personality disorder)

49 Investigations in patients with acute and chronic confusional states

1   A, E, I
2   B, E
3   L

SECTION 3:
CRITICAL REVIEW PAPER

16 FORMAT OF THE CRITICAL REVIEW PAPER

The critical review paper consists of two questions (A and B). Candidates are required to answer all parts of both questions.

Question A

In Question A a condensed form of a published paper is presented followed by questions about the findings of the paper, the study design, methodology and the importance of the paper to clinical practice. There are seven questions (each worth 10 marks) each having further subquestions. The marks for the subquestions vary from 1 to 5.

Question B

In Question B a shorter research study is presented. Usually this is related to the contents of the paper presented in Question A. There are three questions (each worth 10 marks) with subquestions with marks varying from 2 to 5. Most of the questions are concerned with evidence-based medicine.

17 HOW TO PREPARE FOR THE CRITICAL REVIEW PAPER

Candidates should have working knowledge about research methodology and be able to apply this knowledge when evaluating published research.

Core knowledge

Candidates should have an understanding of the following:

- study design and methodology and their applicability to a given published paper
- key features and common sources of problems or biases
- different types of research settings: randomized controlled trials, cohort studies, case–control studies, single-case studies, meta-analyses, systematic reviews, studies involving economic analyses, qualitative studies
- basic statistical concepts (e.g. confidence intervals and probability), and common parametric (e.g. t tests, analysis of variance, multiple regression) and non-parametric (chi-square test, Mann–Whitney U test) tests
- definition and meaning of measures that are important in critical appraisal, e.g. relative and absolute risk reduction, sensitivity, specificity, likelihood ratio, odds ratio, number needed to treat or harm.

A list of commonly used statistical terms and concepts is provided in the Appendix at the end of the book.

Core skills

Candidates should be able to:

- determine the reliability and validity of information and results of a given scientific paper
- determine the clinical significance and relevance of results of a given scientific paper
- detect errors in design and methodology that render the stated conclusions invalid or have an effect on their impact
- understand and assess logically the process and results of critical appraisal of a scientific paper
- provide suggestions for further studies that would confirm or expand understanding in the field under investigation

- place the results of a scientific paper in clinical context and assess how far clinical practice might be changed as a consequence.

Preparation

Candidates should practise applying the above listed skills by discussing relevant published scientific papers in journal clubs and study groups for at least six months before the examination. It is strongly advised that while practising, candidates bear in mind the following framework of questions for all relevant research methodologies. Both questions A and B are designed to test candidates' knowledge and skills along the line of these questions. However, remember that this list is only a guide and does not include all of the questions which can appear in this paper.

NB: '*n*' will be a number (1, 2, 3, etc.) in the actual question.

- What is the name of the study? Define it.
- List '*n*' features of the design of the study and describe how they should help minimize bias.
- List '*n*' potential or actual strengths and/or weaknesses of the design or implementation of the study. For each point listed, explain how it might affect the outcome of the study.
- Give definitions of the outcomes in the study.
- List the features of the sample which might affect the generalizability of the study to all patients with 'X' disease/disorder.
- How do you think the results of this study might affect the management of your patients?
- Give '*n*' reasons why you would consider switching drug A for drug B.
- List '*n*' main findings of the study/tables/figures, etc.
- Summarize '*n*' main conclusions from the table/figure/graph, etc.
- Give '*n*' reasons for exercising caution in applying the results of this study to your patients.
- Describe observations that tend to increase/decrease your confidence in the conclusions of the study.
- Give the advantages/disadvantages of meta-analyses/systematic reviews in comparison with a new large randomized controlled trial.
- How might the study design be altered to overcome disadvantages in a given study?
- Describe methods used to assess methodological quality.

18 HOW TO TACKLE THE CRITICAL REVIEW PAPER

Candidates will find the following tips helpful when attempting the critical review paper.

- Read the questions before reading the presented paper as the questions will give clues about the type of the paper and the difficulties it may pose.
- Try to answer Question B first. It carries 30 marks and it is generally considered easier than Question A, which carries 70 marks. In other words, try to 'bank' as many marks as possible in the first 15–20 minutes.
- Make rough notes before answering each question. This allows one to gather one's thoughts about the study and the subject of the investigation.
- The questions usually have two to five parts/subquestions. It is therefore useful to re-read every question to ensure that nothing has been missed.
- Candidates should pace their time according to the demand/marks allotted to each question. For example, if a question carries 2 or 3 marks, there is no point in spending more than 1 or 2 minutes on it. If a question has three parts with 4, 4 and 2 marks each, it will probably require less time than another question with five parts with 2 marks each.
- Although questions tend to appear in a sequence, candidates should choose the order in which they wish to answer them – beginning with questions they can answer fully and leaving the others for later.
- Give ONLY the required number of answers. For example, if a question asks for five advantages of a study design and a candidate gives six or seven, marks will only be awarded for correct answers among the first five. In other words, incorrect answers among the first five will not be awarded any marks and even if answer 6 or 7 is correct, it will not attract any marks.
- Pay attention to the wording of questions and structure answers accordingly. For example, if the question asks to 'list' advantages, use words or short phrases. If the question asks to 'discuss', use sentences and short paragraphs. If it asks to 'compare and contrast', do both.
- Try to answer all questions as it will enhance the chances of achieving the pass mark.

19 RESEARCH METHODS AND STUDY DESIGNS USED IN PSYCHIATRY

This chapter gives an overview of the topics listed below. It will help candidates to revise the main aspects of these topics and to deal with the questions in the critical review paper of the examination.

- Descriptive observational studies (purely descriptive and only suitable for hypothesis generation)
  - Case reports
  - Case series
  - Cross-sectional surveys
  - Audits
  - Qualitative studies
  - Surveys, e.g. two-phase epidemiological surveys, cross-sectional studies (e.g. ecological or correlational study)
- Analytic observational studies (suitable for hypothesis testing)
  - Case–control studies
  - Cohort studies (controls are not required)
- Experimental studies (causation can be inferred)
  - Uncontrolled or open trials
  - Controlled trials, e.g. randomized controlled trials
- Economic analysis
- Other methods
  - Meta-analyses
  - Systematic reviews

Descriptive observational studies

Case report and case series

Definition

These are either a description of one case (case report) or a number of cases (series). They are actually descriptions of personal clinical experiences. Case reports/series are a most basic form of evidence-based medicine (grade IV). The patients tend to be opportunistically identified from a single location and hence are unrepresentative.

Strengths

- They can disprove some conventional ideas or previous research findings.
- They can bring out a question that can stimulate further research.
- They arise from clinical practice.
- They may have important general implications.
- Quick and easy to do.

Limitations

This type of study has numerous problems:

- It is influenced by all sorts of bias.
- One report does not prove anything.
- It does not give a holistic or complete picture of the issue under question.
- Apparent associations seen may be due to coincidence.
- Non-systematic retrospective study.
- The results can be regarded as unreliable due to misdiagnosis, measurement error and confounding.

Alternative studies

To make the finding of a case report or case series more evidence based, case–control studies or cohort studies could be done in the later stage.

Cross-sectional studies

Definition

It is a study of a given population in a specific time period.

Purpose

- To measure the prevalence of a disorder.
- To identify associations between disease and aetiological factors or risk factors.
- If done twice incidence can be studied.
- Repeated cross-sectional surveys can tell about trends over time.
- To make comparisons between populations or different regions.
- To plan a service.

Study design

A population is screened for both exposure and outcome. The cases can then be compared with those without exposure and conclusions drawn.

The study starts with the selection of a target population, then a sample is taken and case definition devised. The case-ascertainment is completed by applying the case definition to the sample and performing the analysis to estimate the prevalence rate.

Strengths

- Cheap and safe to do.
- Simple to perform.
- Ethical.

Limitations

- One cannot establish causation, only association can be inferred.
- Prone to both selection and information bias.
- Reverse causality can be a problem.
- Confounders can be unequally distributed.

Alternative studies

- Cohort study
- Case–control study.

Sources of bias

Selection bias: For example, while surveying patient satisfaction with inpatient services, bias can be introduced if dissatisfied patients refuse to participate in the study.

Information bias: knowledge of the exposure (disease) may lead the interviewer to introduce a bias while looking for outcome. The interviewer may selectively look for the expected outcome (expectation bias) It can be minimized by:

- blinding the interviewer to the exposure status
- keeping the interviewers unaware of the study hypothesis
- using structured and objective questionnaires (outcome measures).

Critical appraisal of a cross-sectional study (for the study of diagnosis)

Validity

- Was there an independent, blind comparison with a reference (gold?) standard for the diagnosis?
- Was the diagnostic test applied to an appropriate spectrum of patients? (Applied to a range of patients with early and late disease, mild and severe disease, etc.)

Outcome

What is sensitivity, specificity, likelihood ratio, positive predictive value, negative predictive value and the prevalence (pretest probability)?

Applicability

- Is the test available in the given setting?
- Is it affordable
- Is it precise?

- Can one generate a sensible estimate of the pretest probability (prevalence of the disorder in the population before the test is applied)
- Will the post-test probability (prevalence of the disorder in those who test positive on the test) affect the management of a given patient.

Audits

Definition
Audit is the systematic and critical analysis of current practice, comparing it with the generally accepted gold standard.

Purpose
To improve the current practice (medical/nursing/any other).

Study design
Identify the current practice to monitor

Find out the gold standard (from the literature search)

Monitor/compare the current practice with the gold standard

Evaluate the differences

Find out the reasons for the differences

Make recommendation for improvement

Monitor the implementation of recommendations

Re-audit the practice over and again after recommended time periods to identify adherence

The whole process is called 'audit loop'.

Strengths
- It can monitor any aspect of the clinical care cycle, e.g. structure, process, outcome, etc.
- If done with appropriate standards, it improves the quality of clinical care and patient satisfaction.
- It helps to identify inappropriate services and malpractice.
- It acts as a safe guard.

Limitations
- Uncontrolled study.
- Gold standard can differ from place to place.

- Results/recommendations are not universally acceptable as its applicability is very local. To make it usable in a specific situation, the audit should be done in that particular situation.

Critical appraisal of an audit

- Find out what issue a particular audit is going to monitor.
- Think whether it is a clinically significant issue.
- Find out how the gold standard has been set. (National Institute for Clinical Excellence (NICE) guidelines are acceptable. Arbitrary standards are not good and there should be some references available of previous research.)
- Check the number of cases included.
- Check the potential sources of bias: selection bias is most important to look for.
- Find out the actual recommendation and re-audit results.
- An audit does not hold good value without a re-audit.

Qualitative studies

Definition

These studies measure people's subjective experiences, feelings, attitudes, values, etc. to generate ideas and hypotheses.

Methods

Semi-structured interviews, in focus groups and/or through observation. 'Purposive sampling' is done to derive representative samples with desirable demographic characteristics.

Delphi or Delphic process and Nominal group (expert panel) technique: both these approaches require the initial definition of a problem and the selection of 'experts'. They use questionnaires which elicit responses to a range of therapeutic options, which participants rate anonymously. The participants then receive feedback on how their responses compare with that of the group. They are then given opportunities to change their initial response, until consensus is achieved.

Strengths

- These studies offer insight where research is not well established or conventional theories seem inadequate.
- They have validity, provided they are well-conducted.
- They can inform and improve quantitative research.

Limitations

- They are prone to researcher's bias in the collection and analysis of data.
- Without direct observations of the participants, attitudes do not necessarily equate to behaviour.
- They may lack reliability, particularly if only one rater analyses the responses.

Surveys

Two-phase epidemiological surveys

These use screening questionnaires, then interview the participants.

Cross-sectional studies

These studies simultaneously ascertain the presence or absence of disease and the presence or absence of an exposure at one particular point in time. They measure rate, i.e. incidence or prevalence of the disease. Their strength is that they identify patterns of disease. Their limitation is that they cannot distinguish cause and effect.

Ecological or correlational study
These measure associations of disease and are a type of cross-sectional study. In this study, routinely collected data on disease rates are compared with data on the general level of exposure between particular geographical regions. Their strength is that they use pre-recorded data. Their limitation is that they describe populations rather than individuals.

Analytic observational studies

Case–control studies

Definition

Cross-sectional retrospective comparative study to determine the causation/aetiology of diseases. The comparison is done between cases and equivalent controls based on the frequency of presence of attributes of the suspected cause.

Purpose

To identify the aetiology of the disease.

Design

- Cross-sectional
- Retrospective
- Comparative

Strengths

- Less time consuming/inexpensive.
- Suitable for rare diseases.
- Can measure the single disease with multiple risk factors.
- Can evaluate distant and multiple exposures.

Limitations

- Prone to recall bias and selection bias.
- Chances of reverse causality.
- Unsuitable for rare exposures.
- Cannot calculate incidence rate.

Critical appraisal of a case–control study

- Identify the hypothesis/null hypothesis.
- Identify the diagnostic criteria for diseases.
- Check how inter-rater reliability was assured.
- Check comparability of controls with patients, i.e. proper matching and drawn from equivalent population.
- Cases may be filtered, e.g. attended in accident and emergency, which is prone to selection bias.
- Blinding of data gatherers to case or control status or at least to the main hypothesis of the study.
- Any sources of recall bias.
- Address confounding factors, either in the design or during analysis.
- An overly matched control group can obscure the aetiology.
- Statistical analysis is similar as for a cohort study: assess relative risk and its confidence interval.

Cohort studies

Definition

Subjects having a certain condition and/or receiving a particular treatment are followed over time and are compared with another group that is not affected by the condition under investigation. A *cohort* is any group of individuals who are linked in some way or who have experienced the same significant life event within a given period. A cohort could be a:

- Exposure cohort – individuals assembled as a group based on some common exposure (for example exposure to rubella in childhood while studying the aetiology of autistic spectrum disorders).
- Birth cohort (for example, all those born between 1990 and 2000).
- Inception cohort – all individuals assembled at a given point of time based on common factors, e.g. place where they live, education, employment, etc.

Thus, a group with an exposure and a group without exposure in question are followed up over a period of time and the outcomes compared. For example, to find the association between conduct disorder (CD) and antisocial personality disorder (ASPD), a cohort of children with CD (exposure) is followed to see who develops ASPD (outcome). The association can be ascertained by comparing a cohort with an exposure (CD) to a cohort without the exposure (non-CD children) or by making comparison within a cohort.

Purpose

There are two main purposes of cohort studies.

1   Descriptive (to study the frequency): to find the incidence of an outcome or to study the life history of a disease. They are useful to study the prognosis of any condition. Thus, a cohort of patients with schizophrenia can be followed longitudinally to look at their outcome and/or prognosis.

2   Analytical (measure of association): they can be used to analyse the association between the outcomes and the risk factors or predictive factors. They can look at the aetiological factors.

Study design

A cohort can be a:

- prospective cohort – subjects followed forwards in time from the time of the commencement of the study
- retrospective cohort – subjects followed forwards in time from the time of exposure which has happened in the past and then traced forward. For example, in studying the association between CD and ASPD, instead of following the children with CD, one can retrospectively determine a cohort of children who had CD through data from child and family clinics. Then identify how many of these have ASPD. This is quicker and cheaper.

Alternative studies

- Case–control study
- Randomized controlled study

Strengths

- Temporal sequence between exposure and outcome can be studied.
- Rare exposures can be studied.
- Multiple outcomes can be looked at.
- Reverse causality unlikely.
- Bias less likely.

Limitations

- Can be time consuming and expensive.
- There can be substantial attrition rate. Differential loss between those exposed and unexposed can result in bias.
- If a very long follow-up, the hypothesis or question at the beginning of the study may not be of interest at the completion of the study.
- Over time, the exposure status may change.
- Usually restricted to study of one exposure.
- Generally unsuitable for study of rare outcome.

Sources of bias

There can be selection bias, which can be minimized by:

- clear and unambiguous definition of the exposure
- minimize loss during follow-up
- both exposed and non-exposed similar in all aspects except exposure.

Critical appraisal of a cohort study

Validity
- Was a well-defined sample used as a cohort?
- Were the patients followed sufficiently long?
- Was the outcome measure objectively stated at the beginning to avoid bias?
- If a control group was used, was it group matched with the cohort (on parameters other than the exposure)?

Outcome
- What is the relative risk?
- Is the P value and confidence interval stated for the findings?

Applicability
- Were the patients in the cohort similar to a given patient?
- Will the evidence influence doctors' decisions about what they will inform or offer their patients?

Experimental studies

Uncontrolled or open trials

Definition

Subjects receive a treatment, and they are aware of it. These studies are a means of establishing whether a treatment works at all and what sort of adverse effects are present. They are therefore useful in early stages of drug development.

Strengths

Cheap and easy.

Limitations

The absence of a control group means that some or even all of the apparent effects could be attributed to many different sources of bias and other causes, such as the type of patient, severity of disease, a true treatment effect, placebo effect. They overestimate the therapeutic benefits by an average of 20 per cent.

Controlled trials

Definition

In these trials, the experimental group is given the new treatment and 'controls' are given a placebo or standard treatment. They can be open, single-blind, double-blind or triple-blind (i.e. the outcome assessors do not know what treatment the patients had received).

Strength

Relatively straightforward.

Limitations

- No randomization.
- They tend to overestimate therapeutic benefit by about 30 per cent.
- The patients getting new treatment tend to be selected (consciously or not) to have a slightly less severe illness and/or better prognosis.

Randomized controlled trials

These trials include random allocation of treatment in all groups. There is even distribution of both the known and more importantly unknown confounders (e.g. age, sex, prognostic factors) of the therapeutic effects in the treatment groups.

- Strengths: Randomization reduces selection bias and confounding.
- Limitations: Expensive and time consuming.

Cluster trials

These are a type of randomized controlled trial in which subjects are randomized in groups or clusters rather individuals.

- Strengths: useful in evaluating more global aspects of health services rather than one particular treatment as allocation of individual subjects is not possible.
- Limitations: often difficult to find enough clusters to give adequate power. The unit of randomization should be the unit of analysis, which requires a large a number of clusters.

Cross-over trials

In these trials, all participants receive two or more interventions, one after the other, with two groups receiving a different treatment first.

- Strengths: can study treatment of rare chronic disorders. These studies are useful if there are potential ethical concerns, which can arise if one of the treatments is placebo.
- Limitations: historical controls, order effects, carryover effects. Difficulties in ensuring that the trial is long enough to ensure therapeutic effects are manifest in a reasonable number of participants.

Pragmatic trials

These are a type of randomized controlled trial. They have bigger samples with broad entry criteria; the interventions can be feasibly provided as part of routine health care and the outcome is a major clinical event.

Economic analysis

Definition

It is a set of quantitative methods used to compare alternative strategies with respect to use of resources and expected outcome.

Types

Cost minimization

In this method, only the inputs are compared and no outcome measure is taken into consideration. It is used when the effects of both interventions are assumed to be identical, e.g. comparing two drugs by comparing their costs assuming that both are equally effective and have the same bioequivalence.

Cost benefit

In this method input and outputs are measured in monetary terms. Monetary unit is used when one needs to compare the cost of an intervention for one condition with the cost of an intervention for a different condition, e.g. to fund a new electroconvulsive therapy (ECT) machine or to fund clozapine treatment.

Cost effectiveness

This is used when the outcome is measured in terms of natural units – for example, life years gained. For both the interventions, outcome is measured in life years gained. This analysis is used when the effects of intervention can be expressed in terms of one variable. For example, comparing two drugs for a fatal condition. It measures productive efficiency; however, it cannot compare different outcomes.

Cost utility

This is used when comparing the cost of a more effective but more expensive intervention with a less effective but also less expensive intervention. It takes both the quantitative and the qualitative aspects into account. The output measure is quality-adjusted life years (QALYs). The QALY is defined as the number of life years gained and the quality of those years for that individual. The QALY:

* is a measure of outcome in cost utility analysis
* takes into account the number of years gained and also the quality of those years to that individual

- is calculated by multiplying the preference value for that health state with the time the individual is likely to spend in that state (preferred value × the time the individual is going to spend).

Both productive and allocative efficiency is measured. The problem with this method can be in assigning values to different health states, which can be subjective. Moreover, the use of QALYs works in favour of the young rather than the old as QALY equals to health state preference value × time spent in that state.

Health state preference values can be assigned by:

- Rating scale measurements – on a scale between health and death the individual is asked to mark where they would put the state in question. For example, Nottingham Health Profile, SF-16 GHQ, McMaster Health Utilities index questionnaire.
- Time trade-off measurements – how many years of the remaining full health are they willing to sacrifice to be cured of this condition.
- Standard gamble measurements – the respondent is asked to consider the choice between living in the same health state or take a gamble with the intervention giving the odds of success to death if it fails. Odds are then varied to see at which point they consider that the gamble is not worth taking.

A better measure is HYE (health years equivalent), which takes into account an individual's likely improvement/deterioration in the health state in future.

Cost consequence analysis

This is a type of economic analysis where the outcome is measured in terms of its different natural units so that the individuals can assign their own value to a particular state before calculating whether the intervention is worth.

Advantages

Allows health state preference values both for individuals and society to change with time.

It allows analysis to be used as different society/group, from one on which the original 1-1 study was done.

Opportunity costs

This is the lack of resources to do something else. The use of resources in one way means that one has to let go the other interventions and the benefits of the other interventions are foregone. This makes it important to clearly and explicitly define the alternative source of interventions.

Costs

- *Direct* – hospital bills/cost of medicines/travelling/administrations, etc.
- *Indirect costs* – the impact of the intervention on the patient's ability to work (loss of productivity) and their contribution to the nation's productivity.

- *Intangible costs* – these include discomfort, pain, suffering and social stigma, the psychological effect of having, e.g. a scar after operation. It also takes into account the cost shifted to the third party.
- *Incremental cost* – one needs to consider this when comparing a less effective and cheaper intervention with a more expensive and more effective intervention. It is the total extra amount one has to pay to achieve an outcome, over what one would have achieved by giving a cheaper but less effective drug to all the patients.

League table

This is a table comparing costs per QALY gained for different interventions. It indicates the cost to gain one additional QALY.

Critical appraisal of economic analysis

- Validity?
- Have the courses of action been compared?
  - are they appropriate and well defined? Sometimes no intervention may need to be taken into account. Comparing clozapine with haloperidol will be less appropriate than comparing clozapine with olanzapine.
  - are they accurate enough, assuming that the outcome is valued, e.g. randomized controlled trial or meta-analysis used? Judging the effectiveness of olanzapine from a survey may not be appropriate.
- Is it the right type of analysis?
- What is the type of analysis used and what is the outcome measure? Is there any problem with the use of this outcome measure?
- Have the various costs been taken into account?
- Whose perspective is it:
  - the hospital's
  - the government's
  - the society's
  - a drug company's?
- Has a sensitivity analysis been performed?
- Is it here and now or is the future taken into account?
- When the costs/benefits of an intervention are likely to occur in future, their value should be discounted. Most analyses use a figure of approximately 5 per cent.

Other methods

Meta-analyses

Definition
A meta-analysis is the statistical analysis of the results of several studies that are considered combinable by the analyst, taking their weights and precision into account.

Purpose
Meta-analyses allow the results of various studies to be combined in a scientific way. A meta-analysis of randomized controlled trials is the most robust evidence in the hierarchy of the grading system for clinical research.

Strengths
- Several small studies can be combined and the sample size increased.
- As the necessary sample size is reached, even small effects can be detected or excluded which otherwise could not have been possible with a single study.
- If numbers of trials in different populations have similar results, the results can be generalized to all those populations.
- Increases statistical power.

Limitations
- The outcome is limited by the qualities of the primary studies. (What goes in decides what comes out.)
- Studies may be too heterogeneous for the data to be pooled.
- One of the important components of a systematic review and meta-analysis is the publication and location bias.

Combining various trials in meta-analysis
Assigning weights to the trial:

Weights in meta-analysis are based on the standard error of the study. While assigning weights, the following should be considered:

- Methodology – extent to which the design and conduct is likely to prevent the occurrence of systematic errors.
- Precision – this is the measure of the likelihood of random error (width of confidence interval).
- External validity – the extent to which the results can be generalized to the target population. (Internal validity refers both to how well the study was conducted and how confidently one can conclude that the change in the dependent variable was produced solely by the independent variable and not by extraneous ones.)

Weighing can be done by:

- Fixed effect modelling – each study is an estimate of a single underlying effect.
- Random effect modelling – preferred methods as studies are considered true random samples of all the studies. It gives more weight to larger studies with larger sample size.

Systematic reviews

Definition

The comprehensive review of the literature, using prespecified criteria.

Purpose

When a vast amount of research has been done on any particular topic it is difficult to keep up with all this information. Moreover, the results of the studies are often contradictory, making it difficult to practise evidence-based medicine. Systematic reviews provide unbiased summaries of all the studies. They bring a large number of studies together which can be compared and analysed (meta-analysis).

Strengths

- Large amount of information can be assimilated quickly.
- Explicit methods in identifying and rejecting the studies limit the bias, making the conclusions more reliable.
- Results between various studies can be compared to establish their generalizability.
- If inconsistency in the results is present, it can be identified and new hypotheses can be generated about the subgroups.

Limitations

- The outcome is limited by the qualities of the primary studies. (What goes in decides what comes out.)
- Studies may be too heterogeneous for the data to be pooled and compared.
- One of the important components of a systematic review is locating the studies. Bias while locating the studies can affect the outcome of the systematic review. Similarly, publication bias needs to be considered.

Sources of bias

- Publication bias – studies with a positive result or a significant result are more likely to be published.
- Location bias:
  - Language bias, e.g. meta-analyses published in the English language are usually based on studies published in English language journals.
  - Database bias – is bias that arises in databases while including the studies.

For example, only 2 per cent of the articles included in Medline are from the third world countries.
- Citation bias – is introduced if one locates for relevant studies rather than searching the full database. This may result in identifying studies which are supportive and can result in bias.
- Multiple publication bias – studies with a positive result may be used for multiple publications in different journals. This can result in overestimation of the treatment effect.

Steps in the systematic review

1 Set the objectives of the review and select the eligibility criteria.
2 Search for trials using various databases and other resources.
3 Tabulate the results of each study in a standard format to allow comparison between studies.
4 Combine the data, taking into account the weight of each study.
5 Test for heterogeneity.
6 Analyse the results. If the endpoint is binary (disease/no disease) calculate the odds ratio or relative risk. If the data are continuous (weight/blood pressure) calculate the effect size.

Various sources of studies
- Medline
- Cochrane Controlled Trial Register.
- Other databases – Embase, Psychlit
- Foreign language literature
- Grey literature (thesis, reports)
- Unpublished data known to experts in the speciality (personal communications)
- Raw data from published trials.

Critical appraisal of a systematic review

1 Is there a clearly focused question which is clinically relevant? A focused question is necessary as one needs to make a dichotomous decision whether to include the study in the systematic review or reject it.
2 Does the review include the right type of studies? Do these studies address the question asked and do they have an appropriate study design?
3 Did the reviewers try to identify all the relevant studies? Look at which databases were searched. Was there personal contact with the experts? Did they look at the unpublished data? Did the reviewers search for non-English language studies? The exact words used while looking for the studies should be mentioned.
4 Was methodological quality of the studies assessed? Did they use a list of criteria, against which to judge each trial? There needs to be a pre-determined strategy to score each study.
5 Has a sensitivity analysis been done? Sensitivity analysis is a statistical procedure to study the uncertainty of a conclusion. It answers 'What if'

questions. It tells whether the conclusion changes if certain parameters are changed. For example: What if studies of low methodological qualities are included? What if unpublished data is excluded? There are three methods to do sensitivity analysis.

- One-way analysis – when one changes a parameter keeping all other parameters constant.
- Extreme scenario analysis – when one changes a parameter to best possible/worst possible scenario, keeping other parameters constant.
- Monte Carlo – changing various parameters in a predetermined range.

6 How are the results presented and what are the main results? How are the results expressed (odds ratio, relative risk, etc.)? How large is the size of the result and is it clinically meaningful? Can one summarize the result in a succinct way?

Heterogeneity and homogeneity

Studies are said to be *heterogeneous* when the results of various studies differ more than can be accounted by chance. It means that there were methodological differences between the studies and/or there were distinct subgroups of patients.

Studies are said to be *homogeneous* when the differences in the results between the studies can be explained by chance alone.

Heterogeneity and homogeneity can be estimated by the following methods.

- At a glance: If the horizontal lines on the blobbogram overlap, the studies can be said to be homogeneous and the horizontal lines indicate the confidence interval (see below).
- Using the:
  - chi-squared test
  - z statistic
  - Galbraith plot
  - funnel plot.

If the P value for heterogeneity is less than 0.05, then the studies can be said to be heterogeneous.

For the chi-squared test, the value is usually equal to the degree of freedom (the number of trials in the meta-analysis minus one). If the x^2 value is greater than the degrees of freedom, then the studies are heterogeneous. For example, in a systematic review of 10 studies (degrees of freedom = 9), if the x^2 value is less than 9, no heterogeneity exists.

Funnel plot

This is a scatter plot with a measure of treatment effect such as odds ratio on the X axis and a measure of study size on Y axis.

In the absence of publication bias, small studies will scatter at the bottom and large studies will aggregate at the top, giving an inverted funnel. The inverted funnel can be converted to upright funnel by taking precision (1/ SE) on the Y axis. Asymmetry of the brim will denote heterogeneity.

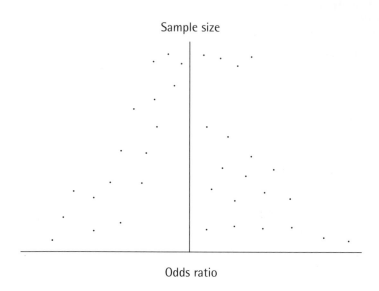

Galbraith plot

This is a graph of z statistics (log odds ratio/standard error) and precision. It tells which study contributes the most to the heterogeneity and gives an idea of the publication bias.

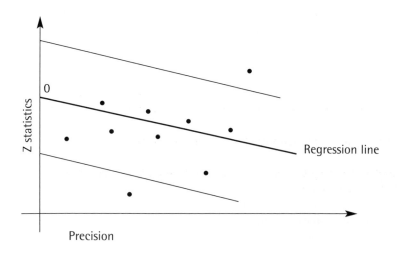

The bold line is called the regression line. The solid line represents the overall log odds ratio and is called the regression line. If publication bias is present the regression line will not pass through 0. If there is no heterogeneity, most of the results will lie between the two lines drawn 2 units above and below the regression line).

Blobbogram

This is also called a forest plot.

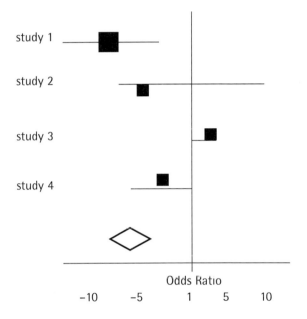

- Each *horizontal line* represents the randomized comparison of individual trials. The width of each line represents the 95 per cent confidence interval (CI). If the CI crosses the vertical line, it means there is no true difference between the two groups in the study.
- The *vertical line* represents the 'line of no effect' and is associated with a relative risk of 1.
- Each *square* represents the point estimate of the effect. This is the most likely value and the results become less likely as they move towards the 95 per cent CI limits.
- The *size of the square* is proportional to the number of the subjects in the study.
- The *diamond* is the weighted average of all the studies. It provides a point estimate with 95 per cent CI.

SECTION 4:
ESSAY PAPER

20 FORMAT OF THE ESSAY PAPER

The essay paper is an important component of the MRCPsych Part II examination. It is also the part most often neglected by some candidates during their preparation for the examination. The paper requires candidates to:

- integrate their knowledge rather than repeat facts
- synthesize diverse information
- develop a reasoned argument
- demonstrate knowledge of relevant literature.

The essay assesses a candidate's ability to put thoughts across succinctly in a legible prose style. It also tests their ability to use their judgement and argue a case in a knowledgeable way. This is important because a psychiatrist's workload includes writing psychiatric reports, complex patient assessment letters, and communicating in a written form on various clinical and management matters.

Format

The paper consists of three questions, of which only ONE question is to be answered. Hence, there is a choice.

There is no division of questions between general adult psychiatry and the psychiatric specialties. Therefore, all three questions will be more wide ranging than in the previous format, with each encompassing aspects of general adult psychiatry and one or more of the specialties. Candidates must read the questions carefully. For example, if the question includes the statement 'throughout the life cycle', it will be necessary for candidates to consider relevant aspects of the question from the perspective of childhood, adulthood and old age. Failure to do so is likely to lead to a poor grade.

21 HOW TO PREPARE FOR THE ESSAY PAPER

The following advice may be helpful in preparing for the essay paper.

- Make a list of the important topics. At least six months before the examination, start making a list of topics most likely to appear in the essay paper. This is obviously pure guess work, but it helps to concentrate one's mind on essay writing.
  - Go through the papers from the last 3–4 years. This should give an indication of the trend for the content of the essay paper.
  - Study topical issues that have been discussed in the relevant scientific journals over the last 12–18 months. See for example, *Advances in Psychiatric Treatment, British Journal of Psychiatry, BMJ*.
  - Go through the latest guidelines published by the Department of Health (www.dh.gov.uk), the National Institute of Clinical Excellence (www.nice.org.uk), the Royal College of Psychiatrists (www.rcpsych.ac.uk), and other relevant organizations.
- Information gathering: once the list is ready, write an essay on one topic at a time. It is generally helpful to write essays on some questions from the past papers, as this will acquaint the candidate with the complexities of the questions. Mere gathering of facts and jotting down points is not sufficient for an essay.
- Refer to standard textbooks for material for the essay. The *New Oxford Textbook of Psychiatry* (Gelder MG, Lopez-Ibor J Jr, Andreasen NC, 2003, Oxford: Oxford University Press) is available free of charge on the internet (go to www.doctors.net.uk).
- Make use of common search engines on the internet to get the latest information on selected topics. For example, while preparing for an essay on suicide prevention in patients with schizophrenia, typing the same words in Google's Advanced search box (with all of the words) will bring up links to many clinical trials assessing the role of clozapine in reducing suicide in these patients.
- Form a study group and seek help from senior colleagues especially in marking the practice essays.

22 HOW TO TACKLE THE ESSAY PAPER

Which essay?

Read the questions carefully and decide which question to answer. It is most unfortunate to change one's mind halfway through writing the essay. Candidates should try to identify the key words in the essay questions and use this as a guide to choosing the essay. See the example below for key words.

Question: Discuss critically the concept of dangerous severe personality disorder, the available treatment options, and the long-term outcome of such problems.

The key words in this essay are 'critically'; 'dangerous severe personality disorder'; 'treatment options'; and 'long-term outcome'.

The rough essay plan

Candidates should spend at least 10 minutes devising a rough plan for the essay on the first page of the answer sheet. This will provide a framework for the essay and will also give the examiner the impression that the candidate has spent time on organizing their thoughts. Furthermore, it allows development of a systematic and logical approach to the structure of the essay and lets the candidate check that all the relevant points have been covered.

Parts of an essay

A well-written essay will have the following distinct components.

Introduction
A good essay starts with an introduction which defines the subject matter and places it in its context.

Main body of the essay
This should state the main themes and develop a discussion of each theme. The candidates should aim to debate both sides of the issue at hand rather than simply present facts.

If asked to make a choice for or against a controversial topic, do not be afraid to do so! For example, in a question such as 'Discuss critically the statement: Cannabis is a dangerous drug and it should remain legally banned in the United Kingdom', candidates should put forward arguments for and against the statement, but then must be able to put forward their choice with reasons rather than just sitting on the fence.

The essay should have a logical sequence and facts should be stated succinctly. Expand on the headings/ideas using biological/psychological/social models; short-term/long-term management plans; local/regional/national initiatives; male/female differences, etc.

Rather than simply writing down all the available information pertaining to the question, candidates should focus on legible writing, proper construction of sentences and the structure of the essay. Write short sentences rather than long ones.

References

It is important to communicate clearly when stating the evidence and developing arguments by referring to studies and the relevant literature. Where appropriate, the research cited should be critically reviewed. To meet the minimum pass mark, it is useful to mention recent and/or relevant articles from journals (*British Journal of Psychiatry*, *Advances in Psychiatric Treatment*, *Psychological Medicine*, etc.).

Conclusion

The essay should end with a succinct conclusion which encapsulates the main points.

23 SAMPLE ESSAYS

1 Pharmacological treatment has been the mainstay of treatment of schizophrenia. Discuss whether psychological therapies have a role in the management of schizophrenia. Give the evidence base for various psychological treatments in schizophrenia.

Introduction

Schizophrenia is probably the most debilitating illness, affecting nearly 1 per cent of the population. Despite the advances in pharmacological treatment of schizophrenia, just under half of the patients continue to experience hallucinations and delusions when on medication. Along with this, the side effects of the medication and the affective symptoms often prompt the patients to look for effective alternatives. In treatment-resistant schizophrenia, a lack of response to medication can generate a therapeutic nihilism.

As a result of this, psychological treatments have been developing, more so in the past decade, in the area of cognitive–behavioural interventions. Earlier traditional medical models stressed the Jasperian concept of 'non-understandability of the symptoms'. This carried the implication that psychological treatment will not work. However, recent evidence shows that not only are these treatments effective, but they are also well received. Hence, psychological treatments have a definite place in the management of schizophrenia. I will discuss the following treatments in some detail:

- Family interventions
- Cognitive–behavioural therapy
- Compliance therapy
- Supportive psychotherapy

Family therapy

The need for the family therapy emerged from the concept of expressed emotions. Brown *et al.* (1958) observed that some patients with schizophrenia when discharged to certain environments are more likely to relapse than others. Subsequently, the Camberwell family interview was developed to demonstrate criticism, over-involvement and hostility. Later, Vaughn and Leff (1976) observed that the amount of face-to-face contact played an important role in causing a relapse. More than 35 hours of direct contact with relatives who showed high expressed emotions was predictor of a relapse. When followed over a 9-month period, about 53 per cent of the patients on medication with high expressed emotions relapsed compared with 15 per cent of the patients on medication with low expressed emotion. Following this, a number of evaluators studied the benefits of family intervention.

Tarrier *et al.* (1994) showed that benefits of this approach were apparent up to 8 years after the intervention. A meta-analysis of six published randomized controlled trials showed family intervention, over a period of 9 months, to be superior compared with controls with regard to the relapse rates. Despite these research findings, integration of family intervention in the management of schizophrenia has been minimal. This is probably due to the lack of adequate training and financial constraints.

Cognitive–behavioural therapy

Cognitive–behavioural therapy (CBT) approaches have been effective in both positive and negative symptoms as well as in acute and chronic stages of illness. Kuipers *et al.* (1997) showed the effectiveness of CBT in reducing the symptomatology of schizophrenia. In treatment-resistant schizophrenia, Pinto *et al.* (1999) showed that clozapine with CBT was superior to clozapine and supportive psychotherapy.

For positive symptoms such as hallucinations, a better understanding of their voices, greater acceptability, teaching strategies to deal with the hallucinations and ability to live with them have been used. The strategies aim to normalize these experiences and reframe the voices into explainable and understandable terms. Hence, the anxiety and distress associated with these symptoms are reduced.

For thought disorders, even with unintelligible speech, themes can emerge; hence spending time with a patient is important. The patient has had years of not being understood and being avoided by others. Tape recording a session can help to pick up these themes. Once the themes have been identified the patient is helped to focus on them in a structured way before moving on to problem-solving strategies.

For negative symptoms such as apathy, anhedonia and avolition, behavioural strategies are more helpful than cognitive strategies. Strategies like activity scheduling, rating of mastery and pleasure and social skills training can be used.

Compliance therapy

It is known that nearly half of the patients do not comply with the medication. The problem can be further accentuated by complex drug regimens, attitudinal factors, lack of insight and inadequate follow-up. Kemp *et al.* (1998) conducted one of the few randomized controlled trials of compliance therapy for patients with mental illness. The study showed that compliance therapy led to improvement in insight, medication and compliance with the medication. Vaughn and Leff (1976) showed that patients who refuse treatment during follow up over a 9-month period after discharge from hospital are approximately three times more likely to relapse compared with those who comply. Compliance therapy includes providing information on the medication and uses strategies like motivational interviewing.

Supportive psychotherapy

Supportive psychotherapy is used to relieve distress and help patients to cope with difficulties. It is based on the common factors of psychological treatment such as the therapeutic relationship, listening, emotional release, information and advice, encouraging hope and suggestion.

Other therapies

Behaviour therapies such as token economy have been used in the past and are rarely used now. Psychodynamic approaches have also been used, but there is little evidence for its use, and it has been reported that it may actually worsen the illness.

Conclusion

Owing to the complex biopsychosocial aetiology of schizophrenia, it is understandable that psychosocial interventions have an important place in the management of this condition. These interventions need to be complementary to the pharmacological treatments. Cognitive interventions, family therapy, compliance therapy and supportive psychotherapy have a place in either the management of schizophrenia or prevention of a relapse. These therapies need to be well integrated into the management of the patient.

References

Brown GW, Carstairs GM, Topping GG (1958) Post-hospital adjustment of chronic mental patients. *Lancet* 2, 685–689.

Kuipers E, Garety P, Fowler D *et al.* (1997) London–East Anglia randomized controlled trial of cognitive–behavioural therapy for psychosis. I: Effects of the treatment phase. *Br J Psychiatry* 171, 319–327.

Kemp R, Kirov G, Everitt B *et al.* (1998) Randomized controlled trial of compliance therapy. 18-month follow-up. *Br J Psychiatry* 172, 413–419.

Pinto A, La Pia S, Mennella R *et al.* (1999) Cognitive–behavioural therapy and clozapine for clients with treatment-refractory schizophrenia. *Psychiatr Serv* 50, 901–904.

Tarrier N, Barrowclough C, Porceddu K, Fitzpatrick E (1994) The Salford Family Intervention Project: Relapse of schizophrenia at five and eight years. *Br J Psychiatry* 165, 829–832.

Vaughn C, Leff J (1976) The influence of family and social factors on the course of psychiatric illness. *Br J Psychiatry* 129, 125–137.

2 Personality disorder has divided psychiatrists as a mental illness. Discuss its place as a distinct entity in the current practice of psychiatry.

Introduction

Perhaps no other condition in psychiatry, in recent times, has triggered such a controversy regarding its existence as has personality disorder. This has gained further impetus since the government initiative to refine the current Mental Health Act. Although it is formally established in the current diagnostic classification systems, it is a diagnosis that is disliked by the *patients*. As stated by Prof. Appleby (1988), it is a diagnosis given to patients, which doctors dislike.

Since the early nineteenth century, attempts have been made to draw a distinction between a personality disorder and mental illness. Pinel (1806) described '*mania sans delire*' for people who are prone to aggressive outbursts. Pritchard (1835) used the term 'moral insanity'. Realizing that these people manifest their behaviour in the absence of mental illness, Koch (1891) used the term 'psychopathic inferiority'. However due to the negative connotations of the word inferiority Kraepelin (1915) rephrased it as 'psychopathic personality'. In present day psychiatry, the term personality disorder has been restricted to the narrow boundaries of dissocial personality disorder and borderline personality disorder.

Concept of mental illness

To understand the concept of mental illness and for that matter personality disorders one needs to look at the various aspects of a medical illness – the medical, the sociopolitical (Kendell, 2002) and the legal aspects. Looking at the medical aspect, any illness can be defined as a deviation from normal health or an abnormal phenomenon, which differs from the norm for that species and puts the affected individuals at a biological disadvantage (Cooke and Hart, 2004). Certainly personality disorders can be regarded as deviation from normal personality, putting these individuals at a disadvantage. From a sociopolitical view a disease is better managed by the medical profession than others like the criminal justice system, the church or the social network systems. Doubts have been raised whether personality disorders can be treated and whether they will improve. However there is evidence that more than 50 per cent of individuals with borderline personality disorders show improvement over 10 years (Davidson, 2002). Legally, as per the Mental Health Act 1983, mental illness is not defined. The Act uses the term psychopathic disorder along with mental illness, mental impairment and severe mental impairment.

I will attempt to put forward the factors for and against the existence of personality disorder as a mental illness.

Factors favouring

There is no doubt that personality disorders have been firmly placed in the classification systems for the past several decades. Both the International Classification of Diseases, tenth revision (ICD-10) and the Diagnostic and Statistical

Manual of Mental Disorders, fourth edition (DSM-IV), acknowledge its existence. Academically, we are mainly driven by the criteria in the classification systems that attempt to diagnose the illness as objectively as possible.

Second, as psychiatrists we regularly encounter the constellation of symptoms described as personality disorder. Almost every psychiatrist or trainee can recollect the nights he or she was on call and was asked to evaluate a young patient who presents with self-inflicted lacerations, feeling of emptiness, appearing in a state of crisis and demanding admission.

A term closely linked with the concept of illness is treatment. A treatment alleviates the symptoms of illness or at times cures them. The presence of an effective treatment reconfirms the existence of an illness. In the past, alcohol was supposed to be something that a person chose to consume in spite of being aware of the consequences. Dependence on alcohol was not considered to be an illness. However, with the advent of effective treatment including drugs like disulfiram and acamprosate, its existence as an illness is less doubted. Similarly, numerous effective treatments have come up for personality disorders. Dialect behaviour therapy (Linehan *et al.*, 1994), cognitive–behavioural therapy (Beck, 1976) and cognitive analytical therapy (Ryle, 1990) have been used in the treatment of personality disorders. Therapeutic communities at the Henderson and Cassell hospitals in London deliver treatment to people with personality disorders. Personality disorders may not be completely curable but then, in no other branch of medicine is curability taken as a criterion of illness. Borderline personality disorders show significant improvement over 10–15 years.

Last but not least, nomenclature is a means of communication among clinicians, providing objective criteria for research and helping to identify those who are in need of help and treatment.

Factors against

It is often said that personality disorders exist on a continuum with no cut-off. Most of the mental illnesses have clear onset, which distinguish them from the premorbid state. Schizophrenia usually starts in the late teens and depression in the late thirties or early forties. However, with personality disorder there is no clear time of onset. It is often a continuation of the temperamental factors in childhood. The opponents of the concept of personality disorder argue that personality disorders are not discrete entities and boundaries between personality and personality disorders are blurred. However, so is the case in many mental illnesses like anxiety disorders.

First, it is the societal acceptance of normality that delineates people with personality disorders from people having supposedly normal personality. With time, values of society change and so does the concept of personality disorder.

Second, it is very hard, if not impossible, to find a person having symptoms of only one personality disorder. There is a significant overlap of symptoms between different personality disorders. Rather than having the diagnosis of personality disorder it would be more effective to have a functional analysis of a person (Gunn and Taylor, 1993). Understanding the person under the headings of thinking, feeling, behaviour and interpersonal problems will be more useful in developing tailor-made package care.

The term 'personality disorder' is often used in a pejorative way. It is a term disliked by the patients. Moreover, such patients are often seen only when they are in crisis. Even on the ward they generate strong emotions in people who come in contact with them and staff often reject them. Thus the label of personality disorder puts them at a disadvantage.

Conclusion

Whether personality disorders exist or not as a mental illness, there is no doubt that they constitute a significant number of cases seen by the health services. According to Casey and Tyrer (1990), about 30 per cent of patients attending general practice with psychiatric morbidity have personality disorders. These have a place as a category in the international classification systems and we routinely encounter them in psychiatric practice. The disorders need to be taken seriously and all National Health Service (NHS) trusts should provide services for personality disorders.

References

Beck AT (1976) *Cognitive Therapy and the Emotional Disorders*. New York: Harper & Row.

Casey PR, Tyrer P (1990) Personality disorder and psychiatric illness in general practice. *Br J Psychiatry* 156, 261–265.

Cooke DJ, Hart SD (2004) Personality disorders. In: Johnstone EC, Cunningham Owens DG, Lawrie SM *et al.* (eds). *Companion to Psychiatric Studies*. Edinburgh: Churchill Livingstone.

Davidson SE (2002) Principles of managing people with personality disorder. *Adv Psychiatr Treat* 8, 1–9.

Gunn J, Taylor PJ (1993) Personality disorders. In: Gunn J, Taylor PJ (eds). *Forensic Psychiatry: Clinical, Legal and Ethical Issues*. London: Butterworth Heinemann.

Kendell RE (2002) The distinction between personality disorder and mental illness. *Br J Psychiatry* 180, 110–115.

Koch JLA (1891) *Die Psychopathischen Minder Wertigkeiter*. Ravensburgh: Dorn.

Kraepelin E (1915) *Der Verfolgungswahn der Schwerhorigen. Psychiatrie, Vol 8, Part 4*. Leipzig: Barth.

Lewis G, Appleby L (1988) Personality disorder: the patients psychiatrists dislike. *Br J Psychiatry* 153, 44–49.

Linehan MM, Tulek DA, Heard HL, Armstrong HE (1994) Interpersonal outcome of cognitive behavioural treatment for chronically suicidal borderline patients. *Am J Psychiatry* 151, 1771–1776.

Pinel PC (1806) *A Treatise on Insanity*. Davis DD (trans). Sheffield: Cadell & Davies.
Prichard JC (1835) *A Treatise on Insanity*. London: Sherwood Gilbert and Piper.
Ryle A (1990) *Cognitive Analytic Therapy: Active Participation in Change*. Chichester: Wiley.

3 Reduction in suicide by mentally ill people is one of the targets of the Department of Health. What are the factors that play a role in suicide by inpatients with schizophrenia? Discuss the steps you would take to reduce the suicide attempts among patients with schizophrenia.

Introduction

Suicide is the most unfortunate outcome of any psychiatric disorder. In schizophrenia it is the single most cause of premature death. Between 4 and 13 per cent of schizophrenic patients commit suicide, whereas 25–50 per cent attempt suicide at some time in their life (Meltzer, 2001). The Epidemiological Catchment Area (ECA; Robins and Regier, 1991) study showed that nearly 28 per cent of the patients with schizophrenia attempt suicide.

Suicide reduction has been the target of many government initiatives. The British Government's white paper *Saving Lives: Our Healthier Nation* (Department of Health, 2004) has set the target of reducing the overall rate of suicide in mentally ill people by one fifth by the year 2010. Though not specific to suicides in schizophrenia, *Safety First* (Department of Health, 2001) gives a good insight into the causes and strategies to deal with suicide.

Suicide in schizophrenia: the risk factors

There are certain factors in suicides committed among patients with schizophrenia, which are different from those in suicides by people with major depression.

Demographic factors

Suicides are more common in males compared with females. However, the gap is narrower in patients with schizophrenia with a ratio of 3:2 against the ratio of 4:1 in depression. The risk decreases with advancing age and nearly 70 per cent of suicides in schizophrenia occur before the age of 30. They are more common in educated, socially isolated and unemployed people.

Illness factors

- There is less risk in those with negative symptoms like apathy, alogia and avolition.
- Suspiciousness in the absence of negative symptoms is a high risk factor.
- Only 4 per cent of patients with schizophrenia commit suicide in response to command hallucinations.
- Affective symptoms increase the risk.
- Among the side effects of medications, akathisia has been associated with suicide risk.
- A group of symptoms called threat/control override symptoms (thought insertion, passivity phenomenon, and persecutory ideations) are linked to aggression in schizophrenia.

Other factors

Comorbid conditions (personality disorders, substance use) and violence are associated with increased risk of suicide. De-institutionalization has increased the risk. According to Stephens *et al.* (1999) the rate of suicide in patients with schizophrenia is four times higher than in the era prior to de-institutionalization.

Neurobiological attributes

Keshavan *et al.* (1994) compared the electroencephalographs of suicidal patients with schizophrenia with those of non-suicidal patients having schizophrenia and reported an increased rapid eye movement (REM) activity. Serotonin and 5-hydroxyindoleacetic acid (5-HIAA) levels have been shown to be increased in people who commit suicide.

Prevention of suicide in schizophrenia

- At patient level
- Early detection and treatment of schizophrenia

Suicides in schizophrenia occur early in the course of the disease. Picking up the illness in the 'trema phase' would be ideal, though this is not always possible. Moreover, one needs to differentiate between negative symptoms of schizophrenia and depressive symptoms, as one is associated with high risk while the other is not.

Medication has a role in reducing the risk of suicide in schizophrenia. Control of symptoms like command hallucinations and threat override symptoms that can reduce the risk of suicide. As stated earlier akathisia is associated with increased risk of suicide. Atypical antipsychotics cause less akathisia compared to the typicals. Some studies have shown that clozapine reduces the suicide risk in patients with schizophrenia (Meltzer and Okayli 1995, Meltzer 1998, 2001 and Meltzer *et al.* 2003).

Regular follow-ups and risk assessments (targeting high risk population)

Risk assessment is an imperfect science. However, regular risk assessments need to be carried out. The post-discharge period is a particular vulnerable period for the patient and the risk is said to be high in the first 6 months after discharge. Patients with suicide risk should be followed up within 7 days of discharge. *Safety First* (Department of Health, 2001) mentions that suicide in mentally ill people is associated with a reduction in the services at the final contact point between the patient and the services. Hence, these patients need to be assertively followed and engaged with the services. Patients with schizophrenia with a moderately high suicide risk need to be on an enhanced care programme.

Disengaged patients

Certain patients repeatedly disengage with the services and need to be followed assertively. These patients may be cared for in a better way by the assertive outreach teams. The reasons for non-compliance with treatment should be explored. Cognitive–behavioural therapy for better control of symptoms and compliance therapy (Kemp *et al.*, 1998) to improve compliance should be applied where necessary.

Dealing with comorbidity

A significant number of patients with schizophrenia use alcohol and some use illicit drugs. Alcohol itself is an independent risk factor for suicide. About 25 per cent of suicides taken place under the influence of alcohol (Barraclough *et al.*, 1974). For difficult patients, expertise of the Dual Diagnosis Services should be sought.

Prevention at NHS Trust level

Appropriate and practical documentation policies need to be in place . The risk needs to be documented and communicated and should not be 'lost' in the thickness of the file. There should be ongoing training for staff, particularly in assessment of suicide risk.

Post-incident appraisals and inquiries should be sensitively conducted. The aim should be to prevent similar incidents occurring and to improve the service rather than blaming and fault finding.

Inpatient suicides

About 4 per cent of suicides occur in inpatients units of which about two-thirds occur by hanging. This can be reduced by taking adequate precautions. Wards should have good observation points. Ligature points should be removed and wards should have collapsible curtain rails. Suicides in wards often occur in the evenings and night and more intense observation is required at these times. There should be a clear observation policy in place.

At community level

Non-governmental organizations such as the Samaritans play an important role in providing support to patients with suicidal ideations. One of the ways of reducing the fatality by overdose is to reduce the number of the tablets in a strip and to make fewer tablets available at one time. Small doses of emetics added to non-steroidal anti-inflammatory drugs can induce vomiting when these tablets are taken in large quantities. Suicide points such as bridges and high buildings should be monitored.

Conclusion

Compared with the normal population, the rate of suicide is increased in patients with schizophrenia. It is important to be aware of the demographic factors, illness factors, the psychiatric history and the support systems of a patient while assessing the suicide risk. Suicides in patients with schizophrenia can be reduced by early detection and treatment of schizophrenia, regular follow-up and risk assessments, dealing with comorbidity, and ensuring appropriate protocols are in place at the Trust and the national level.

References

Barraclough B, Bunch J, Nelson B *et al.* (1974) A hundred cases of suicide: clinical aspects. *Br J Psychiatry* **125**, 355–373.

Department of Health (2004) *Saving Lives: Our Healthier Nation.* London: Department of Health.

Department of Health (2001) *Safety First: Five year report of the National Confidential Inquiry into Suicide and Homicide by people with mental illness.* London: Department of Health.

Kemp R, Kirov G, Everitt B *et al.* (1998) Randomised controlled trial of compliance therapy: 18-month follow-up. *Br J Psychiatry* **172**, 413–419.

Keshavan MS, Reynolds CF, Montrose D *et al.* (1994) Sleep and suicidality in psychotic patients. *Acta Psychiatr Scand* **89**, 122–125.

Meltzer HY (1998) Suicide in schizophrenia: risk factors and clozapine treatment. *J Clin Psychiatry* **59** (suppl 3), 15–20.

Meltzer HY (2001) Treatment of suicidality in schizophrenia. *Ann N Y Acad Sci* **932**, 44–58.

Meltzer HY, Okayli G (1995) Reduction of suicidality during clozapine treatment of neuroleptic-resistant schizophrenia: impact on risk-benefit assessment. *Am J Psychiatry* **152**, 183–190.

Meltzer HY, Alphs L, Green AL *et al.* (2003) Clozapine treatment for suicidality in schizophrenia. *Arch Gen Psychiatry* **60**, 82–91.

Robins LN, Regier DA (1991) *Psychiatric Disorders in America.* New York: Free Press, p. 50.

Stephens J, Richard P, McHugh PR (1999) Suicide in patients hospitalized for schizophrenia: 1913–1940. *J Nerv Ment Dis* **187**, 10–14.

SECTION 5: INDIVIDUAL PATIENT ASSESSMENT (IPA)

24 FORMAT OF THE IPA

Candidates are given one hour to examine a patient and five minutes afterwards to organize their thoughts. They are NOT required to hand in any written material to the examiners. There is an interview with the pair of examiners that lasts 30 minutes. Generally the discussion with the examiners will cover all of the following.

Assessment/Case Summary

15 percent marks; 5–7 minutes

This is the candidate's overall view of the patient derived from salient features in the history and findings from the mental state examination. The discussion at this time will also touch on the diagnosis and findings from physical examination of the patient. If the patient does not have any obvious physical signs, questions will be asked about relevant matters, e.g. examining for extrapyramidal side effects in patients receiving antipsychotic drugs, signs of hyperthyroidism in manic or anxious patients, etc.

Differential diagnosis

15 percent marks; 3–5 minutes

This covers a candidate's ability to justify in detail likelihood of diagnoses by using information from case summary and to suggest appropriate investigations to further differentiate the diagnoses.

Observed interview

20 percent marks; 8–10 minutes

The first examiner to examine the candidate will ask the candidate to interview the patient in front of the examiners to elicit details of specific items that are relevant in the history and mental state examination. Usually no more than two items will be covered. The second examiner will remain silent during this time.

Treatment, management and prognosis

30 percent marks; 5–7 minutes

This will include questions on further enquiries and investigations, short- and long-term management, risk assessment, the roles played by other members of the management team, family and carers. When answering questions about prognosis candidates should mention short-term (i.e. for the current episode) and long-term prognosis.

Clarification of case

20 percent marks; 3–5 minutes

This will include a detailed discussion of diagnosis, differential diagnosis, aetiology, and patient's attitude to illness (insight) and its implications. It will also include biological, psychological and social understanding, psychological formulation, relevant collateral information, knowledge of literature and its application to the patient.

25 HOW TO PREPARE FOR THE IPA

In some ways, the clinical examination is neglected in terms of preparation by a large proportion of candidates. Our clinical work involves diagnosing and managing patients as well as dealing with varied clinical scenarios so it is not uncommon for candidates to feel confident, perhaps overly so, about passing the clinical component of the MRCPsych examination. Another reason which can result in poor performance in the clinical component is a lack of preparation due to inadequate time, and perhaps poor training and supervision. There is a tendency for candidates to wait for the results of the written paper before beginning to practise for the clinical examination. This leaves barely two weeks in which to get oneself ready for the last hurdle as a senior house officer.

For many people, this may indeed be the last examination ever to be taken. After the months of work of preparing for the written examination, it would seem unwise if not foolish to approach the clinical component with anything less than the hard work and dedication it requires. Imagine how devastating it will be to pass the written component, only to fail the clinical examination due to inadequate preparation.

When is the best time to begin preparing?

The best time to start preparing for the clinical examination is around the same time as starting to work towards the written component, i.e. six months before the examination. However, the goals and methods of preparation are entirely different. The candidate should aim to tidy up clinical skills, focus on relevant management issues and develop a systematic way of reasoning. As mentioned above, we are assessing and managing patients all the time in our daily practice so all most of us need to do is improve and streamline existing skills.

Tips for preparing for the IPA

- In the months preceding the examination, try to develop a system of obtaining a history that encompasses relevant points while excluding useless information. Try to present these histories in 7–8 minutes. In short, prospective candidates should treat every new patient in the outpatient clinic or inpatient ward as an examination case in terms of taking a history, requesting relevant investigations, performing relevant physical examination and thinking about important management issues.
- Present these cases to the supervising consultant or specialist registrar (who will be familiar with the examination pattern) and discuss them thoroughly.

- Learn the diagnostic criteria for all the common illnesses and try to justify the diagnosis.
- Try to present complicated cases that involve dual diagnosis, forensic histories, rare or unusual symptoms as well as cases from a variety of settings such as open and locked wards, rehabilitation wards, old age wards, learning disability units, etc. This will prepare candidates for most eventualities in the examination as well as allowing them the opportunity to understand different approaches to assessing and managing different patients.
- Another useful practice is to present cases to different consultants. Not all examiners are the same and the kind of questions you will be asked will vary considerably from consultant to consultant.
- Don't neglect the psychological aspects of treatment or the aetiology. Learn the cognitive and behavioural assumptions that underlie the psychopathology in common illnesses. Candidates should consult with their psychology colleagues about psychological formulations if this is a difficult area for them. Work out a management plan that addresses psychological and social issues for each patient seen.

26 HOW TO TACKLE THE IPA

Fundamentals of making a diagnosis

- Candidates should remember that common things occur commonly. Hence it is useful to have a list of common conditions in mind. For example, the commonest disorders are: depressive disorders, alcohol-related problems, bipolar disorder, schizophrenia, somatisation disorder and borderline personality disorder. Conditions encountered less frequently are: panic disorder, phobic disorders, antisocial personality disorder, obsessive-compulsive disorder, dementia, delusional disorder, eating disorder and learning disability.
- In making a diagnosis or drawing up a list of differential diagnoses, it helps to follow a systematic approach.
- Although the candidate may follow the International Classification of Diseases (ICD)-10 as the diagnostic system, it is useful to think in the Diagnostic and Statistical Manual of Mental Disorders (DSM)-IV format of multi-axial classification to make sense of the patient. First, as a general rule in medicine, the aim is to explain the clinical picture by as few diagnoses as possible, hence the importance of arriving at one or two final diagnosis in axis I, in most cases. In addition to an axis I diagnosis, the patient may have a personality disorder or learning disability. Presence of personality disorder or learning disability is usually indicated by features in the history.
- With regard to Axis I diagnosis, the first step is to identify the syndrome or syndromes that best fits the clinical picture that the patient presents with. The areas of concern evident early in the interview with the patient usually include psychosis, mood disorder, irrational anxiety, somatic symptoms, cognitive deficits and substance abuse and social/legal problems. Arranged in the right order, this will form the basis of the differential diagnosis.
- With regard to the order, it is best to follow the traditional diagnostic hierarchy, i.e. organic conditions including dementia and delirium, followed by psychosis, affective disorders, anxiety disorders, somatoform disorders, alcohol and substance misuse and eating disorder. After the identification of the primary syndrome, the next step is to consider various diagnostic categories which could explain the presentation. This would be followed by narrowing down the list of possible diagnoses to one or more disorders which best fit the clinical picture. For example, if the main syndrome is psychosis, the first possibility to consider is an organic psychosis including those induced by substances or medication, or occurring in the context of general medical conditions and intracerebral pathologies. In absence of any clue to such a possibility, the conditions to consider are schizophrenia, schizoaffective disorder, bipolar disorder and depressive disorder with psychotic features and delusional disorders.

- For an affective disorder, the approach would be very similar to that described above. Following the organic possibilities, the next list of conditions to consider would be psychotic disorders with predominant affective features such as bipolar disorder, depressive disorder with psychotic feature and schizoaffective disorder. The next group of conditions to consider would be depressive disorders, dysthymia, and cyclothymia and adjustment disorder.
- For an anxiety disorder, after considering the possible organic conditions, and assuming absence of psychotic features, it would be necessary to exclude a depressive disorder which subsumes most anxiety symptoms. In the next step consider the individual anxiety states/diagnoses and narrow down the choices to one or best fit. For post-traumatic stress disorder (PTSD), the trauma forms the pivot in the presentation followed by the characteristic symptom pattern. For somatic symptoms, the chronological relationship with any depressive symptom becomes important in arriving at the most likely diagnosis. The chronology is also important in establishing the primary diagnosis when psychotic symptoms or mood symptoms coexist with alcohol or drug abuse.
- Candidates should remember that alcohol and drug abuse colour the entire clinical picture, in a similar way as personality disorders and learning disability or borderline intellectual states do. For example, substance abuse could lead to a plethora of symptoms covering the entire range of conditions including psychosis, depression, hypomania and anxiety. In such patients, the context of the symptomatology should give a clue to the underlying condition. Moreover, the life story and/or the psychiatric history in these patients are likely to have gaps, inconsistencies and inexplicable events. Hence it pays to be vigilant for these clues at the beginning of the interview, which shapes the focus and the emphasis of the subsequent interview. Candidates should also remember that substance abuse and personality disorder tend to co-exist.
- If it is not possible to make a definite diagnosis, a list of differential diagnoses must be offered. It is useful to start with a broad basis of possible diagnoses and apply the features of the case to gradually narrow down to one diagnosis if possible. It is important for a candidate to demonstrate to the examiners the thinking and the logic behind the final or preferred diagnosis. In real life, the final diagnosis is informed by collateral information from a variety of sources including the knowledge of the patient's course of illness or treatment and progress during the index admission for inpatients. As candidates do not have the benefit of the collateral information, the considerations shaping the differential diagnostic process are perhaps as important as the final diagnosis itself.

Summarizing the case

Candidates should present salient features, i.e. signs and symptoms as elicited, relevant aspects of family and personal history such as history of mental illness, substance misuse and stressors, main findings of mental state examination indicative of the preferred diagnosis.

Observed interview with the patient

This involves eliciting at least two pieces of information usually from the history or mental state examination. The questions will depend on the diagnosis. It includes taking a piece of history, premorbid personality, forensic history, past psychiatric history, alcohol and drug history, insight, suicide risk, mood, first rank symptoms, manic symptoms, obsessive compulsive symptoms, a range of anxiety symptoms, cognitive functions including frontal lobe functions, judgement, general knowledge, etc.

Classification

Candidates are expected to know the principles of classification, to have a working knowledge of DSM-IV and to have a more detailed knowledge of either ICD-10 or DSM-IV.

DSM-IV Multi-axial classification

- Axis I – Clinical syndromes and 'conditions not attributable to mental disorder' that are the focus of attention and treatment
- Axis II – Personality disorders, mental retardation (learning disability)
- Axis III – Physical disorders and conditions
- Axis IV – Severity of psychosocial stressors
- Axis V – Highest level of adaptive functioning in the last year

Aetiological factors (biological, psychological and social)

Candidates should be able to consider why this patient has developed this disorder at this point in their life, in this particular form and with this particular content to their mental state. They should consider the aetiological factors as follows.

- Predisposing factors, e.g. family history suggestive of genetic loading, and learnt behaviour, social circumstances, organic factors such as alcohol and illicit drugs.
- Precipitating factors, e.g. life events.
- Perpetuating/maintaining factors, e.g. ongoing stress, lack of insight, non-compliance with care plan, comorbidity, substance misuse, primary and secondary gains.

,ortance of psychological factors

ndidates would be expected to be able to give a psychological explanation about their patients. They would also be able to describe some of the different models available with an indication of which model they are employing and why.

Behavioural assessment

The commonest form of behavioural analysis uses the simple ABC model, i.e. Antecedents, Behaviours and Consequences. For example, to what extent:

- has there been faulty early learning
- the current behaviour is being rewarded, and therefore maintained
- avoidance is playing a role in the presentation.

Psychodynamic assessment

This includes:

- early experiences
- current psychological (e.g. ego defence) mechanisms that are being used and the purpose that such mechanisms might appear to have for that individual
- the part that these factors might have played in the genesis and maintenance of the mental disorder.

The interplay between enduring personality traits and current symptomatology is important. Other factors such as primary and secondary gains are important in some patients with somatoform, anxiety, depression, stress-related and dissociative disorders.

Cognitive assessment

This includes:

- Identification of underlying dysfunctional beliefs derived from early learning experiences. Themes (e.g. need for approval, perfectionism) rather than the actual assumptions which might be identified in a single interview.
- Identification of a recent critical incident (if any), that may have activated the underlying belief, e.g. in depression, loss, rejection or failure to attain goals; in anxiety, perceived threats, etc.
- Current symptom profile: (i) either in cognitive (reported automatic thoughts or images), behavioural, affective and biological components (ii) or in the patient identified list; and how (i) and (ii) may relate to underlying beliefs.
- Identification of biases in information processing in terms of the negative cognitive triad (view of self, world and future) and/or a description of the commonest types of distortion shown by the patient (e.g. overgeneralization, all or nothing thinking).

The place of physical examination in the clinical examination

A physical assessment is made by a series of observations and physical examination of the patient. It is mandatory in the clinical examination. It is important for the initiation of investigations and management of physical symptoms, thus avoiding unnecessary referrals to other specialists. If a candidate cannot complete the physical assessment for whatever reasons, they must be prepared to justify such omissions to the examiners. They should also be prepared to discuss what further observations and investigations would be appropriate.

The physical examination is important for the following reasons:

- It is essential to appraise accurately the physical signs and symptoms associated with a primary mental disorder.
- It provides a basis for informing and if necessary reassuring patients about their physical health.
- It enables the psychiatrist to be satisfied that there is no physical illness present that either aetiologically or fortuitously is related to the mental disorder.
- It enables the psychiatrist to remain competent in physical examination of patients and also to check the findings of other doctors.
- It enables the psychiatrist to make appropriate referrals to other specialists.

Further reading

Morrison J, Munoz RA (1996) *Boarding Time: A Psychiatry Candidate's guide to Part II of the ABPN examination*, 2nd edition. Washington DC: American Psychiatric Press.

27 COMMONLY ENCOUNTERED CLINICAL SITUATIONS

The aim of this chapter is not to provide a complete list of knowledge and skills required in this section of the examination but to serve as a guide to the most commonly encountered clinical situations.

Schizophrenia

Differential diagnosis

- Bipolar affective disorder
- Schizoaffective disorder
- Drug-induced states
- Depression with psychotic symptoms
- Obsessive-compulsive disorder
- Alcoholic hallucinosis
- Organic syndromes, e.g. temporal lobe epilepsy
- Personality disorder, e.g. borderline personality disorder (emotionally unstable personality disorder)

Aetiology

Genetic factors

Monogenic theory (single-gene models), polygenic theory (cumulative effect of several genes), genetic heterogeneity theory (schizophrenia is a group of disorders of different genetic make-up or perhaps with genetic and non-genetic forms).

There is an average lifetime risk of about 5–10 per cent among first-degree relatives of patients with schizophrenia compared with 0.2–0.6 per cent among first-degree relatives of controls indicating a familial aetiology which combines the genetic element and effects of the family environment. Twin and adoption studies point to a definite genetic basis.

Environmental/developmental factors

- Intrauterine events (e.g. birth complications, prenatal exposure to influenza, and winter births).
- Neurodevelopmental antecedents, e.g. childhood cognitive and social impairments.

Drug misuse as a cause of schizophrenia

The relative risk of 2.5 times greater in individuals who use cannabis and six times greater in heavy users of cannabis.

Biochemical theories

The dopamine hypothesis (pre-synaptic dopamine release is increased in acute psychosis, and increased dopamine release cannot account for the symptoms of chronic schizophrenia), role of serotonin (allelic variation in the 5-hydroxytryptamine 2a ($5\text{-}HT_{2a}$) gene is a risk factor) and glutamate (a major excitatory and neurotoxic neurotransmitter).

Dynamic and interpersonal factors

* Psychodynamic theories
  - According to Freud, in the first stage, libido is withdrawn from external objects and attached to the ego. The result is exaggerated self-importance, Since the withdrawal of libido makes the external world meaningless, the person attempts to restore meaning by developing abnormal beliefs and fantasies.
  - According to Melanie Klein, the origins of schizophrenia are in infancy. She also believed that in the 'paranoid position' the infant deals with innate aggressive impulses by splitting both its own ego and the mother's representation into two incompatible parts, one wholly bad and the other wholly good. Only later does the child realize that the same person can be bad and good at different times. Klein further advanced the theory that failure to pass through this stage adequately was the basis for the later development of schizophrenia.
* The family as a cause of schizophrenia: This includes concepts of 'schizophrenogenic' mother, marital skew (one parent yields to the other's (usually the mother's) eccentricities, which dominate the family), and marital schism (the parents maintain contrary views so that the child has divided loyalties). Recent investigations into these theories have not confirmed them. It is now believed that the abnormalities in the parents could be an expression of genetic causes or secondary to the disorder in the patient. Expressed emotions play an important role in psychotic relapse rather than the origin of psychosis, high expressed emotions increasing the risk of relapse two to threefold.

Social factors

* Culture: The incidence rates of schizophrenia are remarkably similar in widely different places (Jablensky, 2000) with possible exceptions in northern Sweden and Slovenia.
* Occupation and social class: Patients with schizophrenia are more likely to have been born into socially deprived households.
* Migration: High rates of schizophrenia have been reported among some migrants. Harrison *et al.* (1988) have reported an incidence of about 6 in 1000

in Afro-Caribbeans particularly in the 'second generation' born the UK. In contrast, rates in the Caribbean are not appreciably increased.

- Psychosocial stressors, e.g. life events and difficulties, may act as precipitants of schizophrenia.

Schizoaffective disorder

Differential diagnosis

Same as in schizophrenia. See above.

Aetiology

Similar to schizophrenia, the first-degree relatives have an increased risk of both mood disorders and schizophrenia.

Persistent delusional disorders

Differential diagnosis

- Schizophrenia
- Paranoid personality disorder
- Schizotypal disorder
- Pathological/morbid jealousy

Aetiology

There is an increase in the rate of delusional disorder in first-degree relatives of patients with schizophrenia. However, relatives of patients with delusional disorder do not have an increased risk of schizophrenia or schizotypal disorder. This familial association pattern has been called *asymmetric co-aggregation* which may be due to a number of factors.

There seems to be a familial association between alcoholism and delusional disorder. There are inconsistent reports of association with polymorphism in the gene for the dopamine D_4 receptor.

Depressive disorder and dysthymia

Differential diagnosis

- Normal sadness
- Anxiety disorders, e.g. generalized anxiety disorder, phobic anxiety disorders, obsessive compulsive disorder, mixed anxiety depressive disorder

- Bipolar affective disorder
- Schizophrenia
- Drug-induced states
- Dementia and other organic causes, e.g. carcinoma, infections, diabetes, thyroid disorder, Addison's disease, systemic lupus erythematosus
- Alcohol abuse/dependence

Aetiology

- Genetics: Life time risk of 20–30 per cent in first-degree relatives, likely to result from the combined effect of modest or even small effect, so called polygenic inheritance.
- Personality: Most relevant personality features are perfectionist traits and anxiety.
- Early environment: Parental discord/separation.
- Vulnerability factors and life difficulties/events.
- Brown (1958) identified three vulnerability factors: having to care for young children, not working outside the home, and no confiding relationships.
- Psychological theories:
  - Freud suggested that just as mourning results from loss by death, so melancholia from loss of other kinds. He also proposed that the depressed patient regresses to the oral stage at which sadistic feelings are powerful and problems at this stage somehow predispose to depression in later life.
  - Melanie Klein suggested that if the stage of 'depressive position' is not passed through successfully, the child will be more likely to develop depression when faced with loss in adult life.
  - Beck proposed that depressed patients have negative thoughts/depressive cognitions. They consist of automatic thoughts that reveal negative views of the self, world, and the future which are sustained by cognitive distortions, i.e. illogical ways of thinking (arbitrary inference, selective abstraction, overgeneralization and personalization).
- Neurobiological approaches:
  - Monoamine hypothesis. This suggests that depressive disorder is due to an abnormality in a monoamine neurotransmitter system (5-HT, noradrenaline, and dopamine) at one or more sites in the brain.
  - Endocrine abnormalities. Depression is common in Cushing's syndrome, Addison's disease, hypothyroidism and hyperthyroidism. There seem to be abnormalities at various points in the hypothalamic–pituitary–adrenal axis. Dexamethasone non-suppression is more common in the depressed patient with melancholia.
  - Immune system. There is growing evidence that patients with depression manifest a variety of disturbances of immune function. Cytokines may have a direct role in provoking mood disorders.

Bipolar affective disorder

NB: Bipolar I – in which mania has occurred on at least one occasion; Bipolar II – in which hypomania has occurred but not mania.

Differential diagnosis

- Schizophrenia
- Schizoaffective disorder
- Drug-induced states (amphetamine and other illicit drugs)
- Depressive disorder
- Organic brain disease involving frontal lobes, brain tumour and human immunodeficiency virus (HIV) infection

Aetiology

- Genetics: Life time risk of 20–30 per cent in first-degree relatives
- Neurobiological approaches: There may be a heightened responsivity to increased dopamine neurotransmission in patients at risk of mania but it is unlikely to be due to increased presynaptic dopamine release.

Generalized anxiety disorder

Differential diagnosis

- Panic disorder
- Depressive disorder
- Mixed anxiety and depressive disorder
- Schizophrenia
- Substance misuse, especially alcohol or drug withdrawal symptoms
- Dementia
- Physical causes, e.g. thyrotoxicosis, phaeochromocytoma, hypoglycaemia, and hyperventilation

Aetiology

- Genetics: Life time risk of about 19.5 per cent in first-degree relatives of probands.
- Stressful events: It often begins in relation to stressful events, and some cases become chronic when stressful problems persist.
- Adverse childhood experiences.
- Psychodynamic theories: Anxiety arises from intra-psychic conflict which occurs when the ego is overwhelmed by excitation from any of three sources:
  - the outside world (realistic anxiety)
  - the instinctual levels of the id, including love, anger and sex (neurotic anxiety)
  - the super ego (moral anxiety).

- Cognitive–behavioural theories:
  - Conditioning theories propose that anxiety arises when there is an inherited predisposition to excessive response of the autonomic nervous system, together with generalization of the responses through conditioning of anxiety to previously neutral stimuli.
  - Cognitive theories propose that it arises as a result of a tendency to worry unproductively about problems and to focus attention on potentially threatening circumstances.
- Personality: Anxiety as a symptom is associated with neuroticism. It is associated with anxious personality traits, anxious-avoidant personality disorder and also other personality disorders.
- Neurobiological mechanisms: Complex mechanisms involving several brain systems and several neurotransmitters are involved.

Panic disorder

Differential diagnosis

- Generalized anxiety disorder
- Phobic anxiety disorders, especially agoraphobia
- Depressive disorder
- Substance misuse, especially alcohol or drug withdrawal symptoms
- Acute organic brain disorder
- Physical illnesses: Thyrotoxicosis, phaeochromocytoma, hyperventilation, mitral valve prolapse

Aetiology

- Genetics: 30–40 per cent inherited vulnerability.
- Biological causes:
  - Abnormalities in presynaptic alpha-adrenoreceptors that normally restrain the activity of presynaptic neurones in the areas of the brain concerned with the control of anxiety.
  - An abnormality of benzodiazepine or 5-HT receptor function.

Phobic anxiety disorders

Specific phobia

Differential diagnosis

Diagnosis is seldom difficult as the patients are open about their problems.

- Depressive disorder
- Obsessive-compulsive disorder

Aetiology

- Persistence of childhood fears.
- Genetic factors: A modest genetic vulnerability combined with phobia-specific stressful events.
- Psychoanalytic theories: Phobias are not related to the obvious external stimulus but to an internal source of anxiety. This external source is excluded from consciousness by repression and attached to the object by displacement.
- Cognitive–behavioural theories: According to conditioning theory, a specific phobia arises through association learning and/or observational learning. Cognitive factors include fearful anticipation of phobic situations and selective attention to phobic stimuli.
- Prepared learning: This refers to an innate predisposition to develop persistent fear responses to certain stimuli.
- Cerebral localization: Significant changes in blood flow were observed in paralimbic structures, visual association areas and thalamus in some positron emission tomography studies.

Social phobia/social anxiety disorder

Differential diagnosis

- Generalized anxiety disorder
- Depressive disorder
- Schizophrenia
- Avoidant personality disorder
- Body dysmorphic disorder
- Social inadequacy

Aetiology

- Genetics: Social phobias are commoner in relatives of probands than in the general population.
- Conditioning: Conditioning and learning seem to play an important role.
- Cognitive factors: The principal cognitive factor is an undue concern that other people will be critical. This is often called a 'fear of negative evaluation'. It is not known whether this cognition precedes the disorder or develops with it.

8.3 Agoraphobia

Differential diagnosis

- Social phobia
- Generalized anxiety disorder
- Depressive disorder
- Delusional disorders

Aetiology

Onset of agoraphobia

- Cognitive hypothesis: It proposes that the anxiety attack develops because the person is unreasonably afraid of some aspect of the situation or certain physical symptoms experienced by chance in the situation.
- Biological theory: It proposes that the initial anxiety attack results from chance environment stimuli acting on a person who is constitutionally disposed to respond with anxiety.
- Psychoanalytic theory: It proposes that the initial anxiety is caused by unconscious mental conflicts related to unacceptable sexual or aggressive impulses which are triggered indirectly by the original situation.

Maintenance of agoraphobia

- Learning theories: Conditioning could account for association of anxiety with more and more situations and avoidance learning could account for the subsequent avoidance of these situations.
- Personality factors: People who are dependent and prone to avoid rather than confront problems often develop agoraphobia.
- Family factors: It could be maintained by family problems and overprotective attitudes of other family members.

Obsessive compulsive disorder

Differential diagnosis

- Generalized anxiety disorder
- Panic disorder
- Phobic anxiety disorder, e.g. agoraphobia, social phobia
- Depressive disorder
- Schizophrenia
- Organic cerebral disorders

Aetiology

- Genetics: It is found in about 5–7 per cent of the parents of patients.
- Organic brain disorders:
  - Patients with Gilles de la Tourette's syndrome have obsessional symptoms. In one study, 70 per cent of patients with Sydenham's chorea were reported to have obsessive-compulsive symptoms (Swedo *et al.* 1994).
  - Brain imaging studies which are not wholly consistent, suggest abnormalities in the orbitofrontal cortex, anterior cingulate, and parts of basal ganglia and thalamus.
  - There is an uncertainty as to whether 5-HT function is abnormal in these patients in spite of the fact that obsessive-compulsive symptoms respond to selective serotonin reuptake inhibitor (SSRI) drugs.

- Early experience: It is uncertain whether early life experiences play a part in the aetiology of this disorder. However, mothers with the disorder might be expected to transmit symptoms to their children by imitative learning.
- Psychoanalytical theories:
  - Freud originally suggested that obsessional symptoms result from unconscious impulses of an aggressive or sexual nature. These impulses could potentially cause extreme anxiety, but it is reduced by the action of the ego defence mechanisms of repression and reaction formation.
  - Freud also proposed that the person regresses to the anal stage of development as a way of avoiding impulses related to the subsequent genital and Oedipal stages.
- Learning theory: According to this theory, obsessional rituals are the equivalents of avoidance responses. However, a general explanation of this idea cannot be sustained because anxiety increases rather than decreases after some rituals.
- Cognitive theory: It proposes that it is not the occurrence of intrusive thoughts that has to be explained but the patient's inability to control them. The patients respond to the thoughts as if they were responsible for their consequences, for example, harm to other people.

Conversion disorder (DSM-IV)/dissociative disorder (ICD-10)

Diagnosis

In practice, the diagnosis of these conditions can be difficult because it requires:

- establishing that the loss of function is not a result of an identifiable neurological or other physical disease
- consideration of psychological factors usually in the form of a psychological trauma or conflict, and
- differentiating them from malingering symptoms.

There is no real way of differentiating conscious from unconscious processes. The test that is often used is that of consistency.

Differential diagnosis

- Neurological conditions, e.g. brain tumours
- Somatisation disorder
- Hypochondriasis
- Neurasthenia
- Depressive disorder
- Schizophrenia
- Persistent delusional disorders

Aetiology

- Psychodynamic theories: According to Freud, there is conversion of psychological distress in to physical symptoms with symbolic meaning.
- Cultural expectations.
- Social factors: Social and behavioural factors appear to be major determinants of the onset and development of conversion symptoms.
- Central neuropsychological and neurophysiological mechanisms: Spence (1999) suggested that conversion symptoms are associated with patterns of localized abnormalities of cerebral functions.

Somatization disorder

Differential diagnosis

- Undifferentiated somatoform disorder
- Hypochondriasis
- Body dysmorphic disorder
- Conversion disorder
- Factitious disorder
- Medical functional disorders, e.g. irritable bowel syndrome, hyperventilation syndrome
- Depression
- Generalized anxiety disorder

Aetiology

- It is considered to be a single stable syndrome.
- The interpretation of bodily symptoms is affected by several sets of factors:
  - previous illness and treatment experiences
  - illness beliefs
  - social circumstances
  - personality and mental state.
- The symptoms may be maintained by:
  - behavioural, psychological and emotional consequences which reinforce the underlying perceptions and interpretations
  - peripheral and central neurobiological mechanisms associated with chronic anxiety
  - the reactions of others.

Hypochondriasis

Differential diagnosis

- Somatization disorder
- Other disorders as under somatization disorder above

Aetiology

The cause is unknown. Cognitive theory emphasizes the faulty appraisal of bodily sensations in leading to false beliefs and maintaining psychological reactions and behaviours.

Body dysmorphic disorder

Differential diagnosis

- Hypochondriasis
- Schizophrenia
- Delusional disorder, somatic type
- Depression
- Obsessive compulsive disorder
- Social phobia

Aetiology

The cause is unknown.

Adjustment disorders

Differential diagnosis

- Acute stress disorders
- Depressive disorder
- Generalized anxiety disorder
- Post-traumatic stress disorder (PTSD)

Aetiology

Stressful circumstances are the necessary cause of adjustment disorders. Individual vulnerability is also important.

Post-traumatic stress disorder

Differential diagnosis

- Generalized anxiety disorder
- Depressive disorder
- Phobic anxiety disorders, e.g. panic disorder, agoraphobia
- Acute stress disorders
- Adjustment disorders

Aetiology

The stressor

- Genetic factors: Vulnerability appears to be related to temperament, neuroticism, age (children and old people are more vulnerable), and gender (women are more vulnerable)
- A previous history of psychiatric disorder.
- Previous traumatic experiences including separation from parents and child abuse.
- Pre-existing low self esteem.
- Neuroendocrine factors: These indicate sensitization of noradrenergic and serotonergic systems. Cortisol levels which normally increase in response to stress are reduced in PTSD.
- Psychological factors: Fear conditioning.
- Cognitive theories suggest that PTSD arises when the normal processing of emotionally charged information is overwhelmed, so that memories persist in an unprocessed form in which they can intrude into conscious awareness.
- Psychodynamic theories emphasize the role of previous experiences in determining individual variations in response to severely stressful events/experiences.

Maintaining factors

- Negative appraisals of early symptoms.
- Avoidance of reminders of the traumatic situation (prevents deconditioning and cognitive reappraisal).
- Suppression of anxious thoughts which is known to make them more likely to occur.
- Financial compensation (if applicable).

Personality disorders

Cluster A: paranoid, schizoid, schizotypal
Cluster B: antisocial, borderline, histrionic, narcissistic
Cluster C: avoidant, dependent, obsessive-compulsive

Borderline/emotionally unstable personality disorder

Differential diagnosis

- Antisocial personality disorder
- Histrionic personality disorder
- Paranoid personality disorder
- Generalized anxiety disorder
- Depressive disorder
- Schizophrenia
- Bipolar affective disorder
- Substance misuse

Aetiology

The causes of personality disorder are largely unknown. Genetic factors have been proposed along with various early life experiences.

- Genetic factors: There are conflicting results from studies of prevalence of borderline personality disorder in the relatives of the probands with this disorder. A high rate of affective disorder has been reported in relatives.
- Psychoanalytic theories propose a disturbed relationship with the mother at the stage of individuation of the child.
- Physical and sexual abuse in childhood.

Antisocial/dissocial personality disorder

Differential diagnosis

- Borderline personality disorder
- Paranoid personality disorder
- Narcissistic personality disorder
- Substance misuse

Aetiology

- Genetic factors: These are more important in adults than in antisocial children or adolescents where shared environmental factors are more important.
- Cerebral pathology and cerebral maturation:
  - A kind of prefrontal dysfunction.
  - There is weak evidence of delay in maturation of the brain on electroencephalography.
  - Low levels of the 5-HT metabolite, 5-hydroxyindoleacetic acid (5-HIAA) have been found in the cerebrospinal fluid of individuals who have committed acts of unpremeditated violence. 5-HT-mediated prolactin release is lower in individuals with a history of impulsive aggressiveness.
- Developmental theories:
  - Separation from mother, and parental relationship problems.
  - Social learning in childhood.
  - Growing up in an antisocial family.
  - Lack of consistent rules in the family.
  - A way of overcoming an emotional problem.
  - Poor ability to sustain attention and other impediments to learning.

Eating disorders

Anorexia nervosa (restricting, binge-eating and purging types)

Differential diagnosis

- Bulimia nervosa
- Eating disorder not otherwise specified
- Depression
- Physical illness

Aetiology

- Genetic factors:
  - 6–10 per cent of female siblings of patients suffer from the condition.
  - An association between eating disorders and affective disorders.
- Biological factors:
  - Hypothalamic disturbance has been most frequently cited as the likely biological factor contributing to aetiology. However, the disturbance is similar to that found in starvation due to other causes and it tends to return to normal when the patient regains weight.
  - Several studies have found neuropsychological deficits such as reduced vigilance and attention span, impairment of visuospatial processing and impaired associate learning. Most of these changes return to normal on regaining weight.
  - Brain imaging studies have found significant sulcal widening and/ventricular enlargement which appears reversible on weight gain, but *not* in all patients.
  - Unilateral temporal lobe hypoperfusion has been reported in regional cerebral blood flow radio-isotope studies.
- Social factors: The rate of family dieting, and concerns about shape and weight are increased and also of overt eating disorders.
- Individual psychological factors:
  - Bruch (1974) suggested that these patients are engaged in 'a struggle for control, for a sense of identity and effectiveness with the relentless pursuit of thinness as a final step in this effort.'
  - Crisp (1977) proposed that, whereas anorexia nervosa is at one level a 'weight phobia', the consequent changes in body shape and menstruation can be regarded as regression to childhood and an escape from the emotional problems of adolescence.
  - Fairburn *et al.* (1999) have suggested that the premorbid personality traits of these people equip them poorly for the demands of adolescence.
- Family factors:
  - Minuchin *et al.* (1978) held the view that a specific pattern of relationships could be identified, consisting of enmeshment, over protectiveness, rigidity,

and lack of conflict resolution'. They also suggested that the development of anorexia nervosa in the patient served to prevent dissent within the family.

- Kalucy *et al.* (1977) suggested that the other family members have an unusual interest in food and physical appearance, and the family are unusually close knit to an extent that might impede the child's adolescent development.

Bulimia nervosa

Differential diagnosis

- Anorexia nervosa
- Eating disorder not otherwise specified
- Obesity

Aetiology

- Genetic factors:
  - It appears to be the result of exposure to general risk factors of mental disorder, especially depression and of risk factors for dieting.
  - It remains possible that there is an inherited abnormality in the regulation of weight and eating habits.
- Other factors:
  - Adverse childhood experiences.
  - Perfectionism and low self-esteem.
  - Sexual abuse.

Substance misuse

Alcohol dependence syndrome

Differential diagnosis

This should include consideration of the following comorbid mental disorder:

- Schizophrenia
- Anxiety disorders, especially generalized anxiety disorder, agoraphobia, social phobia, and panic disorder
- Mood disorders, especially depression and bipolar affective disorder
- Neurotic and stress-related disorders, especially PTSD and adjustment disorders
- Obsessive-compulsive disorder
- Eating disorders
- Personality disorders, especially antisocial personality and borderline personality disorders

Aetiology

- Genetic factors:
  - Alcohol use: The liability to lifetime alcohol use is environmentally determined. The risk of illicit, under-age drinking has strong genetic determinants.
  - Alcohol misuse and dependence: It is well established that alcohol dependence aggregates in families. There are two types of alcohol dependence: type 1 and type 2. Type1 alcoholism has a later age of onset and is mildly genetic. Type 2 alcoholism is strongly genetic with an early age of onset. It is associated with criminality and antisocial personality disorder in both adoptee and biological father.
  - The mechanism of genetic transmission is not known, however, it is thought to be biochemical, involving the metabolism of alcohol or its central effects or psychological, involving personality.
- Other biological factors:
  - Abnormalities in alcohol dehydrogenase or in neurotransmitter mechanisms.
  - Abnormal performance on cognitive tasks and on the P300 visual evoked response, which is a measure of visual information processing.
  - Sons of alcohol dependent men are less sensitive to the acute intoxicating effects of alcohol. Presumably, if subjects experience less subjective response to alcohol, they may tend to drink more, thus putting themselves at risk of developing alcohol dependence.
- Learning factors:
  - Alcohol use. It has been proposed that an expectation of positive effects of alcohol in childhood correlates with the degree of subsequent alcohol use.
  - Alcohol dependence. It has been proposed that the combined biochemical and cognitive approaches involve the role of dopamine release in mesolimbic pathways in mediating incentive learning.
- Personality factors such as anxious traits, a pervading feeling of inferiority and antisocial personality disorder.
- Mental disorders such as depressive disorder, panic disorder, social phobia, bipolar disorder and schizophrenia are associated with alcohol misuse.
- Alcohol consumption in society: It is generally agreed that rates of alcohol dependence and alcohol-related disorders are correlated with the general level of alcohol consumption in a society.

Drug misuse and dependence

Diagnosis of drug misuse/dependence is generally straightforward. However, there is a strong association between substance misuse, particularly dependence and psychiatric morbidity (usually called dual diagnosis). The following mental disorders should be considered:

- Personality disorders especially antisocial, borderline, and anxious-avoidant personality disorders
- Depression

- Anxiety disorders, especially generalized anxiety disorder, panic disorder, social phobia and agoraphobia
- Schizophrenia
- Bipolar affective disorder

Aetiology

- Availability of drugs.
- Over the counter drugs.
- Prescribed drugs, e.g. benzodiazepines.
- Illicit drugs.
- Personal factors.
- Associated behaviours include a poor school record, truancy or delinquency.
- Traits such as sensation seeking and impulsivity are also common.
- History of mental illness or personality disorder in the family.
- Adverse social environment.
- Societies which condone drug use have a greater risk of drug misuse.
- Peer pressure.
- Social deprivation such as unemployment and homelessness.
- Neurobiology of drugs, e.g. drugs act as positive reinforcers because they cause positive subjective experiences such as euphoria and reduction in anxiety.

References

Brown GW, Carstairs GM, Topping GG (1958) Post-hospital adjustment of chronic mental patients. *Lancet* 2, 685–89.

Bruch H (1974) *Eating disorder: anorexia nervosa and the person within*. London: Routledge and Kegan Paul.

Crisp AH (1997) Diagnosis and outcome of anorexia nervosa: the St. George's view. *Proc R Soc Med.* **70**, 464–70.

Fairburn CG, Cooper Z, Doll HA, Welch SL (1999). Risk factors for anorexia nervosa. Three integrated case-control comparisons. *Arch Gen Psychiatry* **56**, 468–76.

Harrison G, Owens D, Holton A *et al.* (1988) A prospective study of severe mental disorder in Afro-Caribbean patients. *Psychol Med* **18**, 643–57.

Jablensky A (2000) Epidemiology of schizophrenia. In: Gelder MG, Lopez-Ibor J Jr, Andreasen NC (eds). *New Oxford Textbook of Psychiatry*. Oxford: Oxford University Press.

Kalucy RS, Crisp AH, Harding B (1977) A study of 56 families with anorexia nervosa. *Br J Med Psychol* **50**, 381–95.

Minuchin S, Rosman B, Baker L (1978) *Psychosomatic families: anorexia nervosa in context*. Cambridge, MA: Harvard University Press.

Spence SA (1999) Hysterical paralyses as disorders of action. *Cogn Neuropsychiatry* **4**, 203–26.

Swedo SE, Leonard HL, Kiessling LS (1994) Speculations on antineuronal antibody-mediated neuropsychiatric disorders in childhood. *Pediatrics* **93**, 323–6.

SECTION 6:
PATIENT MANAGEMENT PROBLEMS (PMPs)

28 FORMAT OF PMPs

This part of the MRCPsych Part II Examination is concerned with the management of clinical problems or scenarios candidates are expected to have come across during their training.

Patient management problems (PMPs) consist of three vignettes, each lasting approximately 10 minutes. The examiners will allow approximately equal time for each vignette, reading aloud the vignette at the same time as it is being read by the candidate.

In the first 3–4 minutes the candidate will be encouraged to speak freely, e.g. the opening 'probe' will be 'How will you assess and manage this situation?'. Then the examiners will ask three or four more 'probes' to explore the candidate's skills and knowledge further with regard to each vignette.

29 HOW TO PREPARE FOR PMPs

The vignettes usually cover common and occasionally uncommon clinical problems encountered by the candidates during their basic specialty training, i.e. as a senior house officer. It is expected that most candidates would have dealt with these clinical issues in a variety of settings, e.g. inpatient service, outpatient clinics, accident and emergency departments, general hospital wards, the patient's home, police station, hostels, care/nursing homes, day centres, and reception areas. But remember that a scenario may not always be clinical. Questions may as well cover issues such as managing conflict in a team, difficulties with colleagues, ethical and moral dilemmas, so the ability to think on one's feet is invaluable.

A useful time to practise this is when the candidates are on call. Candidates should think of each referral as a scenario and decide what information they would like to have and how they would proceed with an assessment. Write down the problems in order of importance and think of ways to manage each one. Most PMPs are 'real world' scenarios, so do not be afraid to consider a referral to a tertiary centre, consultation with senior colleagues or searching the literature as part of a hypothetical management plan in appropriate cases.

Candidates should practise PMPs on the topics given under the following headings to ensure that they cover a wide variety of vignettes. The topics are grouped by specialty and other aspects of day to day clinical work. This list is not meant to be exhaustive but a guide to real examination experience.

General adult, social and rehabilitation, community and liaison psychiatry, and substance misuse

- Drug-induced psychotic states; schizophrenia; schizoaffective disorder; *folie a deux*; role of antipsychotic drugs including clozapine; available augmentation strategies
- Bipolar affective disorder; rapid cycling bipolar; role of antimanic drugs/mood stabilizers, especially in patients with renal and thyroid problems
- Depression, especially with psychotic symptoms, dysthymia, recurrent and treatment-resistant types; role of various treatment strategies
- Anxiety disorders, e.g. generalized anxiety disorder, panic disorder, agoraphobia, social phobia, specific phobias, mixed anxiety and depressive disorder, obsessive compulsive disorder
- Stress-related disorders, e.g. post-traumatic stress disorder, stress reactions, adjustment disorders

- Substance misuse, i.e. alcohol and illicit drugs; delirium tremens and other withdrawal states; principles of acute and long-term treatments; morbid jealousy; benzodiazepine dependence
- Physical illness and mental illness, e.g. epilepsy, Parkinson's disease, hypertension, diabetes mellitus, thyroid disorders, Huntington's disease, myocardial infarction, chronic fatigue syndrome, irritable bowel syndrome, unexplained medical symptoms
- Personality disorders, especially antisocial, borderline/emotionally unstable, narcissistic, histrionic personality disorders
- Side effects of antipsychotics including depot injections, mood stabilizers, antidepressants and benzodiazepines; neuroleptic malignant syndrome; serotonergic syndrome
- Perinatal psychiatry, especially depression and anxiety in pregnancy, use of prescribed and illicit drugs during pregnancy and breast feeding; maternity blues; postnatal depression; puerperal psychosis
- Somatoform disorders, especially somatization disorder, hypochondriasis and body dymorphic disorder
- Eating disorders, especially anorexia and bulimia nervosa; how to calculate body mass index (BMI)
- Dissociative states; false memory syndrome; chronic pain disorder
- Sleep disorders, especially chronic insomnia
- Grief reactions, e.g. normal and abnormal/pathological such as prolonged, abnormally intense, delayed, inhibited and distorted grief
- Gender identity disorders, e.g. transsexualism, dual role transvestism
- Disorders of sexual preference, e.g. fetishism (cross dressing), fetishistic transvestism, exhibitionism (indecent exposure), voyeurism, paedophilia, sadomasochism

Old age psychiatry

- Acute and chronic confusional states including Alzheimer's, multi-infarct, frontotemporal and Lewy body dementias
- Elder abuse; self-neglect; depression; late paraphrenia
- Power of attorney including enduring and lasting type; court of protection; Testamentary capacity

Child and adolescent psychiatry

- Delays in development, speech and language
- Emotional disorders such as depression, separation anxiety disorder, school refusal, elective mutism, enuresis and encopresis
- Hyperactivity and attention deficit hyperactivity disorder (ADHD)
- Sexual, emotional and physical abuse, child protection issues, at-risk register, assessment of risk of deliberate self-harm and suicide

- Adjustment disorders associated with insulin-dependent diabetes mellitus (type 1), Gilles de la Tourette's syndrome, epilepsy, and physical disabilities
- Conduct disorders including delinquency

Forensic psychiatry

- Psychiatric reports including fitness to plead, diminished responsibility, *actus rea*, *mens rea*; application of Mental Health Act; disposal of the offenders; responsibilities of the psychiatrists

Learning disability

- All levels of learning disabilities; comorbid mental illnesses such as depression, bipolar affective disorder, anxiety disorders, schizophrenia; dementia
- Epilepsy, Down's syndrome, Asperger's syndrome; autistic spectrum disorders
- Forensic issues such indecent exposure, aggression, violence and petty offences
- Abuse by carers and other people

Physical treatments

- Indications, contraindications; cautions, adverse effects, interactions; monitoring; pros and cons of stopping a particular drug
- Guidelines – National Institute of Health and Clinical Excellence and others
- Antipsychotics especially depot injections, atypicals including clozapine, antimanic drugs (mood stabilizers), antidepressants, benzodiazepines and anti-dementia drugs
- Use of atypical antipsychotic drugs in dementia
- Use of antidepressant drugs in children
- Use of drugs in pregnancy, e.g. antidepressants, antipsychotic depot injections, antimanic drugs, heroin, methadone and other illicit drugs
- Electroconvulsive therapy (ECT)

Treatment strategies

- Acute, maintenance and prophylaxis treatment, e.g. lithium, sodium valproate, semi-sodium valproate, carbamazepine, atypical antipsychotics including clozapine; antidepressants
- Augmentation strategies in depression, bipolar affective disorder and schizophrenia

Psychiatric emergencies

- Threatened aggression and violence, de-escalation
- Rapid tranquillization
- Application of common law and Mental Health Act

Psychological treatments

Theory, practice and methods of:
- Aversion therapy
- Biofeedback
- Cognitive analytic therapy
- Cognitive–behavioural therapy
- Counselling
- Crisis intervention
- Dialectic behaviour therapy
- Dynamic psychotherapy
- Eye movement desensitization and reprocessing
- Family therapy
- Flooding
- Group therapy
- Interpersonal therapy
- Social skills training
- Supportive psychotherapy
- Systematic desensitization

Communications skills

- Breaking bad news
- Explanation to relatives/carers about the illness; investigations; treatment, e.g. antimanic drugs, antipsychotic depot injections, antidepressants, clozapine, anti-dementia drugs, ECT; prognosis; use of Mental Health Act; care plan

Uncommon psychiatric syndromes

- Binswanger disease: A rare form of vascular dementia associated with multiple small infarcts, presenting in fifth and sixth decades. Computed tomography (CT) and magnetic resonance imaging (MRI) reveal periventricular demyelination (including external capsule), markedly enlarged ventricles and subcortical infarcts

- Capgras' syndrome: This is characterized by the delusional belief that people, usually known to the patient, have been replaced by doubles, i.e. other persons who appear to look exactly like them.
- Charles Bonnet syndrome: It is mostly reported in elderly persons, it is characterized by formed, complex, persistent, repetitive and stereotyped visual hallucinations, recognized by the patient as not real. It is not associated with delusional ideas or hallucinations in other modalities.
- Cotard's syndrome: It is characterized by the presence of nihilistic delusional ideation. The delusion tends to recur intermittently, rather than being chronic, and may be a feature of mood disorder, schizophrenia and organic disorders.
- Couvade syndrome: It affects male partners of pregnant women during their pregnancy or at the time of delivery.
- De Clerambault's syndrome: It is characterized by a delusional belief held by the patient (almost invariably female) that a man usually older, of higher status, famous, wealthy or in a professional relationship with the patient, is deeply in love with her.
- Diogenes' syndrome: It is characterized by hoarding of objects, usually of no practical use, leading to the neglect of one's home or environment. It is considered to be a behavioural manifestation of an organic disorder, schizophrenia, depression, obsessive compulsive disorder, or a reaction to life stresses in a certain type of personality.
- Ekbom's syndrome:
  - Restless legs syndrome: It consists of an unpleasant sensation in the lower limbs that tends to be worse in the evening or at night and hence may interfere with sleep, causing insomnia. It can be associated with antipsychotics and benzodiazepine withdrawal.
  - Delusional parasitosis: It is characterized by delusional beliefs that the patient is infested by parasites. It is associated with extremely unpleasant sensation of worms, ants, bugs, mites, or other small insects that are biting and crawling or creeping over or under or burrowing into or out of areas of the skin. It is usually associated with toxic psychoses caused by alcohol, cocaine or morphine, but may be a manifestation of psychotic depression, schizophrenia or dementia.
  - 'Pisa syndrome' or pleurothotonus: It is characterised by tonic reflection of the trunk to one side which may be seen as a form of tardive dystonia, as a side-effect of antipsychotic medication or as a symptom of Alzheimer's disease.
- Fregoli's phenomenon: It is characterised by a delusional belief that strangers are actually people, with whom the patient is familiar, in disguise. In this way the patient believes he or she is being pursued or persecuted.
- Ganser's syndrome: It is characterised by sudden onset and appearance of 'approximate answers', e.g. 2+2= 5, clouding of consciousness, memory disturbance, talking at cross purposes (Vorbeireden) and dissociative symptoms. It has been thought of as a factitious 'simulated' psychosis, schizophrenia, or an acute psychotic reaction, and more recently a dissociative disorder.

- Meige's syndrome: It is an idiopathic movement disorder characterised by blepharospam and oromandibular dystonia. It may be confused with tardive dyskinesia and can occasionally occur as a side-effect of antipsychotic medication.
- Munchausen's syndrome (Asher syndrome): It is a multiple factitious disorder in which patients present, often dramatically, with a variety of physical and or psychiatric symptoms with the aim of being regarded as ill and given medical attention and treatment.
- Othello syndrome: It is characterised by delusional jealousy where the patient believes that his partner is being unfaithful. It may be a symptom of schizophrenia, alcohol dependence, paranoid personality disorder and delusional disorder.

30 HOW TO TACKLE PMPs

Patient management problems can be daunting. A PMP is best thought of in terms of a real-life situation. Most of us know how to handle simple and complex scenarios that arise in our clinical practice. The difficulty lies in trying to translate this ability into words that will present a coherent and comprehensive action plan in the examination.

The most important aspect of answering a PMP is structuring the answers while prioritizing the issues that arise. With a basic structure in the background the candidate will ensure that nothing is left out. Prioritizing issues enables the candidate to address each aspect of the problem in order of its importance, and thus present a coherent and well thought out management plan.

An example of structuring is as follows: think of information required before an assessment; how and where the assessment will be carried out; what specific areas should the assessment concentrate on; where would the patient be managed in the short term and subsequently the long term. With regard to prioritizing, that is addressing the most important issues, an example would be to place emphasis on the safety of children.

The key to success in PMPs is to answer the questions according to the seriousness and the location of the situation, e.g. threatened violence in a reception area, general hospital wards, hostels etc. In some ways, PMPs are like seeing three patients each for the IPA component of the clinical examination. The following framework will help candidates to formulate their answers in a systematic manner.

- Assessment – this includes detailed history taking, collateral information from important sources, mental state examination, and risk assessment. Risk assessment must include:
  - risk to the patient's health (both mental and physical)
  - risk to the safety of the patient by self-neglect, deliberate self-harm, violence from others and suicide
  - risk to the safety of other people
  - risk of serious exploitation
  - risk of inability to seek and organize help
- Possible diagnosis/differential diagnosis
- Relevant investigations/enquiries
- Management usually based on a bio-psycho-social model or other relevant to a given situation, e.g. an emergency
- Discussion of prognosis
- Communication skills
- Ethical issues:
  - Confidentiality
  - Consent
  - Compulsory treatment

- Negligence
- Problems of the doctor–patient relationship
- Children
- Research
- Setting priorities
- Role as a doctor
- Role as a colleague
- Role as a member of society
- Advising people whom one does not know or with whom there is no official link or connection
- Advising mentally ill people about marriage
- Suicide pacts
- Advising employers, colleagues and licensing authorities (e.g. General Medical Council, Driving Licence Authority)

Confidentiality is fundamental to medical practice. Disclosure of information should be kept to a minimum and consent should be obtained. Doctors may be obliged to disclose information, i.e. breach confidentiality to a third party in the public interest (of the community as a whole or a group or individual within the community). The General Medical Council (2000)* states: 'where a disclosure may assist in prevention, detection or prosecution of a serious crime. Serious crimes in this context will put some one at risk of death or serious harm, and will usually be crimes against the person, such as abuse of children.' *General Medical Council (2000) *Confidentiality: protecting, providing information.* London: General Medical Council.

Consent: in general competent persons have a right to refuse medical treatment/ investigations, even if this refusal results in permanent disablement or death. There are several situations in which explicit consent is not needed. The provisions of common law, i.e. acting in the best interest of the patient can be used as follows:

- Implied consent. For example when a patient holds out his arm to have his blood pressure measured.
- Necessity. When a grave harm or death is likely to occur without intervention and there is doubt about the patient's competence.
- Emergency: When it is possible to prevent immediate serious harm to the patient or others, to prevent a crime, or to prevent serious deterioration of the patient's condition.

If the patient does not have the capacity to give or refuse consent, no one else can give proxy consent on behalf of the patient.

Capacity to consent: It depends on the patient's ability to:
- comprehend and retain information about the investigations and/or treatment
- believe this information
- be able to use it to make an informed choice.

31 SAMPLE PMPs

1 General adult psychiatry – ethical issues

The police picked up a 28-year-old dishevelled and unkempt man on a cold winter night. He claimed that he was a psychiatrist SHO at your hospital. The police believe that he was deluded and a danger to himself as well as the public. He is brought to your hospital under Section 136 of the Mental Health Act 1983. On his arrival he threatened to leave the accident and emergency department.

Suggested probes
1   How will you initially assess the situation?
2   You recognize him as your colleague, how will you then proceed further?
3   If you consider that he is in need of inpatient care, discuss how you will arrange this.

Points to be covered
1   Duty of care to the patient whether a colleague or not.
2   Follow the usual psychiatric assessment procedure.
3   Consult the senior medical staff on call and seek their advice.
4   Consider admission to another unit out of the area, if necessary, under a section of the Mental Health Act.
5   Liaise with his immediate family, the clinical director/medical director, or chief executive or the senior manager on call.

2 Substance misuse – possible alcohol abuse

You are called to see a 45-year-old woman in the accident and emergency department who just had a 'panic attack' and fainted while shopping in the town centre. She appears preoccupied with her worries about her daughter's impending wedding. You notice that she smells of alcohol. She denies having a drink problem and explains that she had lunch with one of her friends. On physical examination, you find that she has palmar erythema, a tremor, pale jaundice, tachycardia and enlarged liver.

Suggested probes
1   How do you propose to further assess?
2   Discuss the specific physical investigations.
3   What are the main principles of management?
4   What are the differential diagnoses?

Points to be covered
1   Detailed history from patient as well as informant(s) if possible, especially about excessive drinking.
2   Full blood count, urea and electrolytes, liver function tests, gamma-glutamyl transferase, thyroid function tests, electrocardiogram (ECG), chest X-ray.
3   Detoxification either as an inpatient or outpatient basis depending on the support available. One should consider a course of a serotonin selective reuptake inhibitor in view of the panic attacks. Long-term management should include complete abstinence or controlled drinking with support from substance misuse service and other support groups such as Alcoholics Anonymous.
4   Differential diagnoses: Panic disorder, generalized anxiety disorder, depression, agoraphobia, alcohol dependence syndrome, an attack of syncope.

3 General adult psychiatry – gender issues

A 34-year-old insurance salesman is requesting gender reassignment surgery. He has dressed in women's clothing since childhood, although he stopped this for a short period during the early years of his marriage, which has now ended. He is now in a homosexual relationship. He has decided to seek gender reassignment surgery, recognizing that he has always felt that he was a woman.

Suggested probes
1   What are the important factors to establish in the history for the diagnosis?
2   What are the generically accepted components of assessment?
3   Give an outline of the psychiatric management prior to surgery.

Points to be covered
1   A sense of overwhelming gender dysphoria from an early age:
     –   Early dressing in clothes associated with the opposite gender, a brief stage of fetishistic dressing, i.e. eroticized dressing in adolescence.
     –   Intense distaste or hatred towards sexual organs that the patient currently has.
     –   An intense desire to participate in the stereotypical, culturally normal activities of a woman.
     –   Masturbatory fantasies concerning vaginal penetration.
2   Assessment:
     –   Physical cause e.g. intersex.
     –   Fetishistic cross-dressing (transvestism) may occasionally present in transsexuals.
     –   To exclude a serious mental illness as psychosis with or without depression.
3   Psychiatric management prior to surgery:
     –   Living as a woman for a minimum of 2 years is the real life test required for male to female transsexuals.
     –   Female sex hormones and anti-testosterone agents may be administered during this period.
     –   Various cosmetic procedures such as depilation and creation of secondary sexual characteristics may also precede definitive and irreversible surgery.
     –   Support throughout the transition process that will include matters such as divorce, etc.

4 General adult psychiatry – depression

You are seeing a 40-year-old woman with six children under the age of 15 years in your outpatient clinic. Her husband, who is 15 years senior to her, is unemployed and abuses alcohol. She looks undernourished and feels scared for no apparent reason. She also complains of disturbed sleep for the past 3 months.

Suggested probes
1   How will you assess this patient?
2   Discuss the diagnostic possibilities.
3   Which physical investigations will you consider and why?
4   Discuss the prognostic factors in this case.

Points to be covered
1   Detailed history from the patient and her husband if available. Explore her main worries and problems.
2   Organic/physical illness: Thyrotoxicosis, diabetes mellitus, pulmonary tuberculosis, anaemia, etc.
3   Mental disorders: Depression, generalized anxiety disorder, panic disorder, anorexia nervosa, alcohol abuse/dependence, and benzodiazepine dependence.
4   Physical investigations: Full blood count, erythrocyte sedimentation rate (ESR), urea and electrolytes, thyroid function tests, liver function tests, gamma-glutamyl transferase, serum B_{12} and folate levels, chest X-ray, and electrocardiogram (ECG) to rule out any underlying physical illnesses.
5   Prognostic factors:
     –   Premorbid personality
     –   Diagnosis and comorbidity
     –   Previous psychiatric history
     –   Financial problems
     –   Husband's alcohol problem
     –   Motivation and compliance with treatment
     –   Social support

5 General adult psychiatry – bipolar affective disorder with obsessive compulsive symptoms

A 35-year-old married white mother of five children under the age of 10 years, presents with a long history of bipolar affective disorder and a dislike of sex. She washes all her bed linen and takes a bath after sexual intercourse with her husband. She refuses to take contraceptive measures or consider sterilization on religious grounds. She is now 3 months pregnant and has stopped taking her lithium just after missing her period.

Suggested probes
1   What are the main components of your assessment?
2   How will you counsel her and her husband about the present situation and future pregnancies?
3   Outline the main components of her management.

Points to be covered
1   History of mood swings (stability or lack of it).
2   Ruminations and rituals, reasons for dislike of sex and how she can account for pregnancies so far.
3   Her explanation of religious reasons for not practising safe sex or considering sterilization.
4   Lithium therapy: dose, duration, efficacy.
5   Previous psychiatric history, especially admissions and response to treatment.
6   Was the pregnancy planned or unplanned? What does she want to do about it?
7   Relationship with her husband and family.
8   Counselling should include:
     –   whether she wishes to continue with her pregnancy or not
     –   effects of her pregnancy on her mental state
     –   need for close monitoring
     –   need for lithium or other mood stabilizer, and their effects on the unborn child
     –   possibility of postnatal depression and/or psychosis
     –   whether she would ever wish not to have more children
     –   effects of her illness (relapses/recurrences) on her family, especially the children
     –   effects of pregnancies/child on her own mental health.
9   Management should include:
     –   whether she wishes to continue with her pregnancy or not, and its consequences
     –   regular monitoring
     –   behaviour modification for her rituals
     –   exploration of her dislike of sex, e.g. is it a result of marital problems or vice versa?
     –   selective serotonin reuptake inhibitor drug
     –   marital therapy

- support to look after her five children
- advice about safe sex, sterilization and vasectomy for her husband.

6 General adult psychiatry – urgent management of side effects

A middle aged Asian woman, currently an inpatient for the treatment of paranoid schizophrenia, has experienced difficulties with eating, swallowing and staying still. You are on call and are requested to access her condition. She requests weekend leave. During her examination, you notice rhythmic movements of her lips and tongue.

Suggested probes
1   What steps will you take to assess this patient?
2   What may be your findings?
3   What factors would you consider in granting her request for weekend leave?
4   How will you deal with the situation?

Points to be covered
1   History from the patient and staff about the onset, duration and severity of her condition in relation to the drug therapy:
     –   Duration of drug therapy
     –   Obtain information from the case notes and staff regarding previous history of similar problems and response to treatment
     –   Current drug therapy, type of drug, dosage, route of admission, and its duration
2   Mental state examination
3   Physical examination including gait, muscle tone, reflexes, power, looking for tremors and assessment of physical distress; akathisia, parkinsonism, tardive dyskinesia.
4   Factors to be considered before granting weekend leave:
     –   Current mental state and level of physical distress
     –   Insight
     –   Family support
     –   Whether she is detained under the Mental Health Act 1983 or not. If she is detained under the Act, leave can only be granted by her Responsible Medical Officer, i.e. consultant in charge of her care
5   Depending on her mental state, the pharmacological treatment may include:
     –   reduction or stoppage of her antipsychotic drugs or no change
     –   Addition of an antimuscarinic drug by the intramuscular route, followed by oral administration until further review by the ward team.

7 General adult psychiatry – possible human immunodeficiency virus (HIV) infection

You are asked to urgently see a 27-year-old married man who has become extremely anxious and depressed recently. You find that he has been having a relationship with a 43-year-old man who has recently become unwell. The patient's male partner has had a positive HIV test recently. The patient is afraid he too might have become infected, and he asks for your advice.

Suggested probes
1   How will you deal with this patient?
2   What advice will you give him?
3   How will you manage the patient if he is tested positive for HIV?

Points to be covered
1   Assessment:
–   First determine why the general practitioner wishes to have the man seen urgently, e.g. suicidal risk.
–   Take a full psychiatric history, obtain collateral information and conduct a mental state examination.
–   Clarify if he has a depressive illness or anxiety state, substance misuse.
–   Clarify whether the relationship is sexual or not.
–   He should be advised to have a HIV test with counselling.
–   Advice should be offered concerning his general sexual practices and the question of the patient discussing the matter with his wife should be broached.
–   He must avoid sexual contact with others until he is certain he will not pass the virus on.
2   Management:
–   Patient to discuss the implications of HIV testing with his wife.
–   Regular attendance in HIV clinic to monitor the progress.
–   To treat comorbid mental disorder if necessary.

8 Liaison psychiatry – possible use of Mental Health Act

A 25-year-old female is brought to your local accident and emergency department following an overdose and self-inflicted injuries to her wrists and forearms. She refuses to cooperate with the casualty officer. You are called to assist in this situation.

Suggested probes
1   How will you approach this situation?
2   If she still refuses to be assessed, how will you proceed further?
3   Can you force physical treatment on her?

Points to be covered
1   Obtain whatever information is available about this patient from the casualty staff and other staff if available.
2   Introduce yourself and explain the purpose of your involvement.
3   Acknowledge to the patient that you are aware of her current situation.
4   Ask her to explain why she is refusing to receive treatment and whether she is aware of the consequences of her refusal.
5   Ask her if she is able to discuss reasons for her deliberate self-harm, and recent life events if applicable.
6   Observe her general appearance, behaviour, mood, speech, interaction with staff and other patients (if any).
7   If she still refuses to be assessed on an informal basis, and there are sufficient concerns/uncertainties about her condition, an assessment under the Mental Health Act 1983 should be considered. As she is in a public place, various options are available depending upon the urgency of the situation, e.g. S4, S2 and S136 of England and Wales Mental Health Act 1983. On the other hand, if the clinical impression indicates low or no apparent risk to her health and/or safety, she may be allowed to leave the hospital.
8   Generally speaking no, you cannot force physical treatment on her. However, if her physical injuries are considered due to an underlying mental illness, her detention in hospital for assessment followed by treatment should include physical treatment. Alternatively, she could be treated under the common law, i.e. necessity to treat the patient in her best interests (life and death matters).

9 Liaison psychiatry – disagreement with a colleague

You are seeing a young man in the accident and emergency department. Following your assessment you believe that this patient requires compulsory admission to the psychiatric unit. The approved social worker is of an opinion to the contrary.

Suggested probes
1   What initial steps will you take in this situation?
2   How will you proceed further?
3   If there is still disagreement with your colleague, what will you do next?

Points to be covered
1   Acknowledge the fact that the approved social worker has an equal say in this matter, and is entitled to his/her opinion and can refuse to make an application if not fully satisfied with the medical recommendations.
2   Ask the patient's general practitioner or a s12 approved doctor to examine the patient.
3   Consult your senior medical staff for advice.
4   Seek further clarification from the approved social worker.
5   Seek the views of the patient's nearest relative or next of kin.
6   Reassess the patient and your own opinion.
7   Acknowledge the fact that the approved social worker may be more experienced than you, and that you might be overcautious.
8   If you are still very concerned about the patient, try to persuade him to consider an informal admission.
9   Do nothing more and advise the approved social worker to make the aftercare arrangements if necessary.
10   Arrange a follow-up by the crisis resolution and home treatment or community mental health team according to local protocol.
11   Express your concerns to the patient, carers, general practitioner and senior medical staff and make an entry in their case notes.

10 General adult psychiatry – differential diagnosis of eating disorder

A general practitioner refers a 35-year-old single woman to you. She has a long history of migraine. Over the last 6 months, she has vomited frequently, even without headaches. The general practitioner is worried that she has an eating disorder.

Suggested probes
1   How would you deal with this?
2   What are the possible differential diagnoses?
3   You discover that she had problems with nausea and abdominal pain as a child and failed to sit her A level exams due to her headaches. How will you treat her?

Points to be covered
1   Assessment:
    –   Full history, mental state examination, physical examination and appropriate investigations and obtain collateral information if available.
    –   The general practitioner is worried about an eating disorder – is there any evidence for this, e.g. marked weight loss, abnormal attitudes to food and menstrual irregularities; bulimia and use of laxatives; excessive exercise.
2   Differential diagnoses: If there is little to support an eating disorder, other possibilities are generalized anxiety disorder, depression, dissociative disorder, malingering, unsuspected physical illness, etc.
3   The history (see point 3 above) is supportive of a generalized anxiety disorder. She appears to have had anxiety/neurotic problems for some years. Try to identify why it has become worse, looking at social outlets, job, family and personal relationships; are there any stressors, is there any underlying depression? Treat the condition appropriately.

11 Old age psychiatry – urgent assessment and management of a confused patient

You are asked to see a 69-year-old spinster on a general hospital ward. She was admitted 2 days ago following a mild heart attack and confusional state. She has a history of poorly controlled hypertension and a 20-year history of paranoid schizophrenia. She was found wandering on the street. She stays up late and interferes with her neighbours. She is excitable, irritable and physically aggressive towards staff and other patients.

Suggested probes
1   What steps will you take to assess her condition?
2   If she does not cooperate how will you proceed further?
3   The medics are of the opinion that she does not need any further treatment. They request you to take over her psychiatric care. Outline your plan of action.

Points to be covered
1   Assessment:
   −   Psychiatric history, collateral information, mini-mental state examination.
   −   Study her psychiatric notes, and establish the change in her condition.
   −   Physical examination and basic investigations to rule out common conditions such as diabetes mellitus, urinary and chest infections, etc.
2   If necessary, consider use of the Mental Health Act.
3   Management:
   −   Transfer to a psycho-geriatric bed.
   −   Consider differential diagnoses, e.g. Alzheimer's disease, multi-infarct dementia, toxic confusional state, depression, manic episode of bipolar affective disorder, and relapse of paranoid schizophrenia.
   −   Nursing in a well-lit side room attending to basic needs.
   −   Judicious use of antipsychotics, benzodiazepines and drugs for physical health problems.
   −   Consider her long-term care in a residential care setting.

12 Learning disability – outpatient management of a mentally impaired child

An 11-year-old boy is referred by his general practitioner at the request of his parents. He has been at a school for children who have mild to moderate learning disability for 3 years. He has tuberous sclerosis, a genetic disorder associated with epilepsy. He exhibits a spectrum of behavioural and psychiatric problems. At the last review meeting with the school, the parents were informed that their child was 'unteachable'. Over the last year, he has been reported to have sat in the classroom not paying attention to anything around him, he appeared to be in a world of his own, and he is not making any progress. The school authorities want to send him to a school for children with severe learning disabilities because he is taking up another child's place.

Suggested probes
1   How would you assess this patient?
2   How would you advise the parents on the management of their child?
3   What are the main psychological issues at stake?

Points to be covered
1   Assessment:
    –   Careful and detailed consultation with the parents alone, allowing them to ventilate their feelings.
    –   Assess the child's strengths and weaknesses.
    –   The potential role of the psychiatrist is to liaise with educational and other services to find the best solution for this child's needs.
2   Management. Possible reasons for 'unteachable' child:
    –   Epilepsy and side effects of antiepileptic drugs.
    –   Tuberous sclerosis may affect the child's cognition and behaviour.
    –   Attention deficit hyperactivity disorder (ADHD).
    –   Pervasive developmental disorders.
    –   Factors at school and at home.
    –   Management will depend on the child's strengths and weaknesses, his general level of development and whether he has severe learning disability, attention deficit or pervasive developmental disorders.
    –   Individual educational programmes should be worked out with parents, school and educational psychologists.
3   The parents will experience a range of emotions including guilt, anger and frustration.

13 Forensic psychiatry – psychiatric report

A 59-year-old schizophrenic man with a long forensic history exposed himself to a minor outside her school. You have been asked to see him in prison. How will you assess and manage this case?

Suggested probes
1   How will you assess this patient?
2   What differential diagnoses will you keep in mind while assessing the case?
3   What factors will you consider in the risk assessment?
4   What advice will you give with regard to management if the patient is currently delusional? What will you include in the psychiatric report?

Points to be covered
1   Procedure for assessing someone in the prison which includes making an appointment in advance and mentioning the time you would need with the patient, carrying a form of identification when you visit the prison.
2   Differential diagnoses to keep in mind would be relapse of psychotic symptoms, substance misuse and possibly presenile dementia.
3   Types of exhibitionism, i.e., young person exposing erect penis, masturbating while exposure with previous forensic history and making attempts to contact the victim poses a high risk as compared with an older man exposing flaccid penis while experiencing significant stressful events in his life.
4   Mention that the psychiatric report would include the nature of the index offence, details of sources of information, especially the transcripts of the initial police interview and inmate medical records, history from patient's old notes, community psychiatric nurse and any other person such as the general practitioner or family member, and current mental state. Following that, depending on your findings the recommendations that you would make to the court about further disposal, mentioning a hospital order if required.

14 Child psychiatry – possible sexual abuse

You are seeing a 13-year-old girl in your outpatient clinic in a follow-up appointment. She confides in you that her father comes into her room at night and touches her inappropriately. This has been going on for the past 2 years, and when she told her mother about it, her mother got angry with her and told her not to tell lies. How will you proceed in this situation?

Suggested probes
1   Will you break confidentiality? If so, how will you manage this situation?
2   Will you inform the parents who are in the waiting room about your action?
3   What are the consequences of childhood sexual abuse?

Points to be covered
1   Mention that you might have to ask some questions to get a clear idea of what took place, and would then have to deal with the situation as an emergency, as you cannot allow her to go back with her parents in such a case. You would need immediately to contact the Child Protection Agency, after explaining to the girl that you are legally bound to let them know as her safety is paramount. The session would have to be terminated to prevent contaminating any evidence and everything that the child has said should be clearly documented.
2   Informing the parents would have to come after the child protection agencies are involved, as in this particular case the perpetrator is the father and her mother is not willing to believe it and they might forcibly try to take the child away.
3   The consequences can differ depending on the duration of the child sexual abuse, the amount of coercion and if penetration actually took place. Poor self-esteem can occur along with guilt that in some way the person had encouraged the perpetrator. There can be early sexual behaviour in children. Alcohol and drug use is also quite common. The person would have difficulty in future relationships as well. There is a risk of post-traumatic stress disorder, depression and borderline traits along with repeated deliberate self harm in adult life.

15 General adult psychiatry – ethical issues

A 32-year-old man with a known diagnosis of bipolar disorder, who has been an inpatient for the past 3 months with a relapse of manic symptoms, has been seen to be driving his car around the town. His mood symptoms are currently under control. This information was given to you by his mother, who informs you that while on home leave, he often goes drinking with his friends and drives them around. How will you assess and manage this situation?

Suggested probes
1   What are the risk factors you would look for?
2   What advice would you give the patient?
3   Would you inform the DVLA about the patient?

Points to be covered
1   Mainly current mental state, the quantity that he is drinking, the effect of medication.
2   Does the patient know that he should not be driving? What information would you give him about the DVLA restrictions on driving in such a case?
3   The DVLA advises that driving must cease during the acute illness. Following an isolated episode, re-licensing can be reconsidered when all the following conditions can be satisfied: (i) has remained well and stable for at least 3 months; (ii) complies with treatment; (iii) has regained insight; (iv) is free from adverse effects of medication which would impair driving; and (v) subject to a favourable specialist report.
4   Repeated changes of mood: Hypomania or mania is particularly dangerous with regard to driving when there are repeated changes of mood. Therefore, when there have been four or more episodes of mood swing within the previous 12 months, at least 6 months' stability will be required under condition (i), in addition to satisfying conditions (ii)–(v) above.
5   Mention at what point one would break confidentiality and inform the DVLA. The examining doctor is required to ask the patient to stop driving and encourage him to inform the DVLA. However, if he continues with the offending behaviour, let him know that the doctor is in such a case obliged to let the DVLA know as he is putting other people at risk as well.

16 Substance misuse – alcohol dependence

A 37-year-old married man is referred to you. He has a 10-year history of alcohol-related problems. He presents to the outpatient clinic and says that he would like help with his alcohol problems as it is a constant source of arguments between his wife and him.

Suggested probes
1   How would you establish whether the patient is dependent on alcohol or not?
2   What do you understand by motivational interview?
3   How would you proceed with the management and detoxification?

Points to be covered
1   Awareness of the key points that point to a dependent pattern, especially the Edward and Gross criteria, i.e. increased tolerance, withdrawal symptoms, compulsion, drink seeking behaviour, relief drinking, narrowing of repertoire and reinstatement after abstinence.
2   Motivational interviewing: Awareness of stages of change, i.e., pre-contemplation, contemplation, ready for action, action and maintenance and awareness of intervention by feedback, personal responsibility, advice about cutting down alcohol, menu of alternative options, empathic interviewing and self efficiency.
3   Awareness of situations in which community detoxification is suitable as opposed to inpatient detoxification.
4   Knowledge of different investigations and regimens of detoxification.

17 Substance misuse – heroin abuse

A 23-year-old single woman presents herself to the outpatient clinic. She has been using intravenous heroin for the past 2 years and occasionally also uses cannabis. She has just found out that she is 2 months pregnant and would like help with regard to her drug use. How will you proceed?

Suggested probes
1   What factors do you need to consider in the drug history?
2   What risk factors would you have to keep in mind with regard to management?
3   What significant factors would you need to consider with regard to her social situation?

Points to be covered
1   Detailed drug history to establish a dependent pattern, mentioning harm minimization and relapse prevention.
2   Mention investigations needed, especially with regard to human immunodeficiency virus (HIV) testing as patient is an intravenous drug user.
3   Mention risk factors to the baby post-delivery due to the opiates, and liaison with the obstetric team about the same.
4   Mention risk to the child regarding neglect, abuse, etc. and therefore the type of social support the mother has after delivery.

GLOSSARY OF STATISTICAL TERMS

Analysis of variance (ANOVA)	Used for more than two independent normally distributed samples. It is a parametric statistical test. The test statistic F is the ratio of the between-groups to within-groups variance
Absolute benefit increase (ABI)	Absolute numerical difference between the rates of good outcomes between the experimental and control groups in a study
Absolute risk reduction (ARR)	Control event rates (CER) – experimental event rate (EER). It is the absolute numerical difference between the rates of adverse outcomes in the experimental and control groups in a study
Attributable risk	Also known as the risk difference or absolute excess risk. It is the incidence of the disease in the group exposed to the risk factor being studied, minus the incidence of the disease in the unexposed group
Alpha (α)	Probability of a type 1 error (rejecting a true null hypothesis), i.e. the probability of demonstrating a difference where in fact a true difference does not exist
Berkson's bias	Bias introduced by choosing a non-representative sample
Beta (β)	Possibility of a type 2 error, (falsely accepting the null hypothesis), i.e. the probability of demonstrating no difference where in fact a true difference exists
Bias	Any process at any stage of inference which tends to produce results or conclusions that differ systematically from the truth
Binomial distribution	Said to occur when there are just two alternative outcomes, A or B, for a trial, and a series of trials is carried out. It is a type of discrete distribution in which a set of discrete separate values is taken by a random variable

Bonferroni's correction	Divides the significance level by the number of observations. For example, if five comparisons are being made, the observed P value must be less than 0.05/5 or 0.1 to be at the 0.05 level, but this is regarded as too stringent
Bradford Hill's criteria for causation	Temporal sequence, dose–response relation, strength of association, consistency and biological plausibility
Canonical correlation analysis	A type of multivariate analysis. It may be regarded as an extended form of multivariate regression except that the number of dependent variables is more than one. The canonical correlation is determined and it provides information about interrelationships among the variables
'Ceiling' effect	When the values of many subjects for a variable are near the maximum possible value, it is called 'ceiling' effect. In certain analyses it reduces the possible variation in the sample
Cluster analysis	A multivariate technique that aims to separate coupled data sets into homogeneous categories in the sense that individual members of a given cluster are similar to each other, but different from members of another cluster generated by the analysis
Chi-squared (χ^2) distribution	An asymmetrical distribution. As with t distribution, the shape of the curve varies with different values of the number of degrees of freedom
Chi-squared (χ^2) test	A non-parametric test used to test whether the proportion of people with or without a certain characteristic differs between two or more independent groups
Confidence interval (95 per cent)	Means that the range of values in which one can be 95 per cent confident that the time value of a given population parameter lies
Confounder	A variable associated with both exposure and outcome but not in a causal way

Control event rate (CER)	Risk of outcome event in a control group, i.e. the proportion of people in the control (non-exposed) group of a study who experience a specific event
Control limit theorem	As the sample size increases, the sample mean will approach a normal distribution, no matter what the shape of the parent population is. It is relevant to the interpretation of standard error
Correlation coefficient	A measure of the degree of association between two or more variables. Correlations coefficients range from -1 to $+1$
Cost-benefit analysis	An economic analysis that compares costs and outcomes of two or more therapeutic interventions in monetary terms, e.g. the cost of drugs
Cost-effectiveness analysis	An economic analysis that compares two or more therapeutic interventions in terms of the cost per unit healthcare gain, such as the life years gained or another generic outcome measure
Cost-minimization analysis	An economic analysis in which only the inputs are considered, i.e. the cost of treatment, as the outputs are considered to be equal, e.g. using the cheapest of two equally effective treatments
Cost-utility analysis	An economic analysis that compares two or more treatments in terms of the cost per quality adjusted life year gained. It measures the effects of the treatments on both quality and quantity of life
Cox's proportional hazards regression model	A method of analysing survival data especially when two groups differ in the presence of one or more prognostic factors. It is assumed that the 'relative risk' which is sometimes called the hazard function or ratio is constant. The terms relative risk and hazard ratio though may be similar for specific time points, are not terms which should be used synonymously
Cronbach's α	An index of the internal consistency of a test

Cross-over trials	Patients receive different interventions in turn during the course of the trial
Degrees of freedom (df)	An elusive concept. It is a measure of the number of ways in which a data set may vary. It is usually given by $n-1$
Discriminant analysis	A multivariate technique that allows individual items or people to be separated into different groups according to a given rule or function. It is particularly useful in studies involving psychiatric diagnostic classifications
Ecological fallacy	A spurious association found in an ecological study between an exposure and an outcome at a population level but not at an individual level
Event rate	Proportion of people in whom a given event is observed over a given time period
Experimental event rate (EER)	Risk of outcome event in experimental group, i.e. proportion of people in this group who experience a specific event
Factor analysis	A multivariate statistical technique used to reduce large complex data sets to a smaller number of explanatory variables
Factorial analysis of variance	A multivariate statistical technique that compares the mean of a dependent measure when the sample can be classified in different ways, e.g. age, sex, diagnosis, etc.
F distribution	Related to the χ^2 distribution and is asymmetrical. Tables are available giving the 100 α percentage points, i.e. the value of $F\alpha$ for different numbers of degrees of freedom. The F distribution is used in the analysis of variance when different samples are being compared
F test	A test for the equality of variances of two populations, given by the ration of the between-groups variance to the within-groups variance
Fisher's exact probability test	An alternative to the χ^2 test when the frequencies of each event are small (<5). It allows the determination of exact probability values and uses factorials

Fixed effects analysis	A method used in meta-analysis where two or more studies are combined and there is low heterogeneity
Floating numerator fallacy	For example, it is meaningless to say that there are more patients with bipolar affective disorder in Scotland than England as this compares numerators rather than ratios
'Floor' effect	Where values of many subjects for a variable are near the minimum possible limit, it is called 'floor' effect
Frequency distribution	A systematic way of arranging data. When in the form of a frequency table, the first column gives the possible values of a given variable, which may be categorical or numerical. The adjacent column gives the frequency with which each variable occurs
Galbraith plot	A plot of the standard normal deviate against the reciprocal of the standard error. It is used to investigate heterogeneity but can be adapted to study and quantify publication bias
Generalizability	Refers to the degree to which the findings of a trial can be extended to the general population of eligible persons
Halo effect	Occurs when the subject's responses fit his or her previous responses. It is the tendency of a rater to overestimate a subject's response based on prior assumptions
Hawthorne effect	Non-specific effects caused by the knowledge subjects have that they are participating in an experimental study
Heterogeneity	A term used in meta-analysis where several studies' results differ more than would be expected by chance. Clinical heterogeneity accounts for differences in the population, intervention, control and outcome measures amongst studies. Statistical heterogeneity accounts for statistically significant level of differences between studies in their results
Internal consistency	Refers to whether items on a scale are related to one another or not. Split half, alternate

	form and inter-rater reliability are measures of internal consistency. Cronbach's α is also a measure of internal consistency
Hotelling's T2	A statistical test used in multivariate analysis of variance
Incidence	Rate of occurrence of new cases in a defined population over a given period of time
Incremental analysis	A technique of health economics examining the additional costs that one service or programme imposes over another, compared with the additional effects, benefits or utilities it delivers
Incremental cost effectiveness ratio	A concept used in economic analysis. It is the ratio of the difference in costs to the difference in consequences
Intention-to-treat analysis	An analysis of patients in the group where they were initially assigned irrespective of treatment received. Some of the participants might not have completed the trial. The analysis includes treatment completion and failures to avoid overestimating the benefits of treatment. A method of imputation of outcome, for example last observation carried forward, is required to carry out this analysis
Intention-to-treat analysis based on worst case scenario	Subjects in the treatment arms who drop out are assumed not to have recovered from a disease/disorder. Subjects in the placebo arm (control group) who drop out are assumed to have recovered from a disease/disorder
Kappa (κ)	An index of agreement on a nominal scale. It is given by Po–Pe/1–Pe, where Po is the observed agreement and Pe is the expected agreement.
Kendall's rank correlation	A non-parametric method which gives a coefficient, t (tau) which has the same range as r and r_s: $-1 \leq \tau \leq 1$; $\tau = 1$ implies perfect positive correlation, $\tau = -1$ implies perfect negative correlation
Kruskal–Wallis test	A non-parametric statistical test used for more than two independent samples not normally distributed

Kurtosis	A measure of how far data depart from the standard normal distribution around the mean. Data may be more flattened (platykurtic) or more peaked (leptokurtic)
Last observation carried forward	Dubious for both statistical and clinical reasons. Most patients who drop out of from a trial may do so because of treatment failure and/or side effects. Taking the last observation carried forward may underestimate or overestimate the benefits of the treatment depending upon the treatment or condition being evaluated
Likelihood ratio	Value of a given test result in predicting the presence of disease. Positive = Sensitivity/1–specificity; Negative = 1–sensitivity/Specificity
Likert scale	A scale where a subject is asked to respond to a question by marking one of a series of discrete points in a dimension
Linear regression line	Straight line of best fit on a scatter diagram
Logistic regression analysis	Used to study the influence of several independent variables on dichotomous outcomes
Mann–Whitney U test	Used to compare two populations which are *not* normally distributed. Aims to show difference between two groups in the value of an ordinal, interval or ratio variable
Mean	A measure of central tendency. The arithmetic mean of a set of numbers is the sum of the items divided by the number of items. Others include geometric and harmonic mean
Median	A measure of central tendency and a quantile. It is the middle value of a set of observations ranked in order
Meta-analysis	Weighted average of results from two or more studies. A meta-analysis is often conducted alongside a systematic review. Publication bias is a threat to the validity of a meta-analysis. **Fixed-effects meta-analysis** is used when the results of individual studies

do not show heterogeneity. These assume that there is a single underlying effect and that each individual study is an unbiased estimator of that effect. Fixed effect meta-analysis is a two-step process: the first step is to calculate a common unit of treatment and the second step is to calculate a summary statistic which is a weighted average of the results from individual studies. **Random-effects meta-analysis** is also referred to as DerSimonian and Laird random-effects models. It is used when heterogeneity is present. It does not assume an underlying treatment effect. Effect sizes from individual studies are assumed to be normally distributed. It gives an average treatment effect across studies

Mode

A measure of central tendency. The mode of a set of observations is the value if the observation occurring with the greatest frequency

Multiple regression

A form of regression where one determines the best combination of independent variables to predict a dependent variable

Multivariate analysis

Refers to analysis of statistical data in which there are at least three variates which need to be measured. There are several forms of multivariate analysis used in psychiatric research: canonical correlation analysis; cluster analysis; discriminant analysis; factor analysis; path analysis; principal component analysis; multivariate regression analysis; survival analysis

Multivariate analysis of variance (MANOVA)

A test comparing two or more independent groups on two or more dependent measures

Minimization

Describes a number of ways of allocating patients by taking account of prognostic variables through pre-stratification so that randomization of similar patients is achieved

Multivariate regression analysis

In this analysis, the multiple correlation coefficient is the maximum correlation between the dependent variable and multiple non-random independent variables.

	Assumptions in this analysis include: the dependent variable has a normal distribution, the independent variables have fixed non-random values and random errors in the model have an overall arithmetic mean of zero and normal distribution
N-of-1 trial	A single subject receives two or more treatments sequentially. Can establish effectiveness in an individual patient. It does not involve controls or randomization and is only applicable to certain types of chronic disease
Nominal scale	A measurement scale where numbers are used to represent categories but do not have rank order
Normal (Gaussian) distribution	Has the form of a bell-shaped curve. It is a good approximation to many naturally occurring continuously variable distributions, e.g. height, body mass, white blood cell count, many types of experimental error
Notation	Used to represent the area under the standard normal distribution curve
Null hypothesis	States that there is no difference between the two groups in question and the difference observed is due to chance
Negative predictive value	Proportion of people who score negative in a test who actually do not have the disorder
Number needed to treat (NNT)	NNT = 1/ARR = 1/CER–EER, where ARR = absolute risk reduction; CER = Control event rate; EER= experimental event rate. It is a measure of clinical effectiveness. The number of patients that need to be treated to prevent one bad outcome compared with a control group. The lower values indicate better outcomes. 95 per cent CI should be calculated. It is the inverse of ARR. It can only be compared for treatment for the same condition, for the same therapeutic outcome, over the same period of time and the same controls
Number needed to harm (NNH)	Number of patients who, if they received the experimental treatment, would lead to one

	additional person being harmed compared with the control group. NNH = 1/ARR = 1/EER–CER
Odds	Odds of an event are the number of times the event is likely to occur divided by the number of times it is likely not to occur. In other words, it is the ratio of probabilities of an event happening to its not happening
Odds ratio (OR)	Comparison of the odds of an event happening in one group to that of its happening in another group. OR = Odds of the event in the experimental group/odds of the event in the control group
Ordinal scale	A level of measurement where numbers refer to the rank order of variables, but where the intervals between numbers are not equal, for example social class
Patient expected event rate (PEER)	Rate of events expected in patients who receive no treatment or conventional treatment in the setting of the clinical practice in question
Power (1–β)	Probability of demonstrating a significant difference between two groups where one exists. It is also equal to the probability of not making a type 2 error, i.e. wrongly accepting the null hypothesis when it is false
P value	Probability that the observed results of a study could have occurred by chance. It is also equal to the probability of type 1 error, i.e. wrongly rejecting null hypothesis when it is true
Population	Set of all the people/objects etc., about which information is required
Positive predictive value	Proportion of people who score positive in a test and who actually have the disorder
Paired *t* test	Used for two paired samples or two repeated measures from one sample, which are normally distributed
Pearson's correlation coefficient	A correlation coefficient between two normally distributed continuous variables. Its

significance or confidence interval should always be stated

Proportion
A type of ratio in which the numerator is included in the denominator. The ratio of a part to a whole is expressed as a decimal fraction and it must lie between 0 and 1

Poisson's distribution
Used in situations in which events occur independently and randomly in time or space. Two or more events cannot take place simultaneously; and the mean number of events per given unit of time or space is constant

Pascal's triangle
A triangle of numbers in which each line starts and ends with one, and in which the middle numbers are formed by adding together the two numbers immediately adjacent to it on the line above. Pascal's triangle is useful in situations in which the probability of the two alternative outcomes is equal

Path analysis
A type of multivariate analysis. It uses a series of multiple regression analyses to allow hypothesis of causality between variables to be modelled and tested. Assumptions in using path analysis include: there is a linear relationship between variables, observations are error free and dependent variables are functions of only the variables incorporated in the model and of no others

Principal component analysis
Similar to principal factor analysis and it can be used to try to produce a reduced number of principal components or dimensions from a large number of original variables

Prevalence
Proportion of a defined population that has a disease at a given point in time. There are three subtypes: **Point prevalence** is the proportion of a defined population that has a given disease at a given point in time. **Period prevalence** is the proportion of defined population that has a given disease during a given time interval. **Life time prevalence** is the proportion of a defined population that

	has or had a given disease (at any time during each person's lifetime so far) at a given point in time
Randomization	A process which allows even distribution of both known and unknown confounders (e.g. age, sex, etc.) and avoids the potential selection biases. **Blocked randomization**: Patients are randomized in groups say of six, eight, etc. to ensure that numbers are equal in the two groups. **Constrained randomization**: It ensures that after a certain number of patients has been entered there will be similar proportions in each group. **Stratified randomization**: Patients are allocated on the basis of prognostic variables to ensure that they are evenly distributed, but it requires an additional schedule for each stratum. **Minimization/adaptive randomization**: Each patient is allocated to a particular group by minimizing any differences in important variables as each particular patient is entered into the trial
Randomized controlled trial	A trial in which a group of patients is randomized into an experimental group and a control group. There can be more than two groups in such trials
Range	A measure of dispersion of a distribution. It is the difference between the smallest and largest values in a distribution
Regression analysis	Study of the relation(s) between two or more variables. It is conducted to: (i) know whether any relation between two or more variables actually exists; (ii) understand the relation between these variables; and (iii) predict a variable given the value of others
Reliability	Level of agreement between sets of observations. Types of reliability are as follows. **Test–retest (temporal) reliability**: The level of agreement of observers who are assessing the same material under similar conditions but at two different times. Kappa (κ) is a measure of test–retest reliability. **Intra-rater reliability**: The level of

agreement between assessments by different raters of the same material presented at two or more different times. **Inter-rater reliability**: The level of agreement between assessments made by two or more assessors at roughly the same time. **Split-half reliability**: Characteristically involves dividing a measurement into two halves and using each half to assess the same material under similar circumstances. **Alternate form reliability**: Two supposedly similar forms of measurement used to assess the same material either at the same time or immediately consecutively.

Relative benefit increase (RBI)	The increase in rates of good events, comparing experimental and control patients in a trial as a ratio to the event rate in controls. RBI = EER − CER/CER.
Relative risk (risk ratio, rate ratio)	Ratio of experimental event rate (EER) to the control event rate. For rare diseases, it is roughly equal to the odds ratio.
Relative risk reduction (RRR)	The per cent reduction in events in the experimental group (EER) compared with controls (CER). RRR = (CER − EER)/CER, where CER = control event rate, EER − experimental event rate
Receiver operating characteristic curve (RoC)	A graphical means of assessing the ability of a diagnostic test to discriminate between healthy and diseased individuals
Regression	Prediction of a dependent variable based on its relation with a another independent variable
Regression to mean	Tendency for extreme values on a measure to decrease with repeated measurement or time
Reverse causality	The situation where a disease causes the apparent exposure rather than vice versa. This is particularly likely in case–control and descriptive studies
Risk ratio	Ratio of risk in the treated group (EER) to that in the control group (CER) used in randomized trials and cohort studies

Sample	A representative subset of the given population
Sampling	Process of selecting a sample. There are several types of sampling. **Cluster sampling:** The population is divided into clusters or units which are related, e.g. hospital, wards, etc. It may be multistage or multiphase. **Periodic sampling:** Every nth number of the population is selected. **Probability sampling:** It is a useful way of identifying potential respondents. It relies on the principles of randomization. **Purposive sampling:** A sample is chosen on the basis of particular characteristics. It is used in qualitative research. **Random sampling:** Each member of the population has an equal chance of being selected. **Stratified random sampling:** A given population is first divided into a number of strata. Random samples are then selected from each stratum with the size of each sample chosen usually being proportional to the size of the stratum from which it is selected
Scheffe's *post hoc* test or Tukey's honestly significant difference test	A *post hoc* test most commonly used with an analysis of variance to detect where significant differences lie. It offers a suitable compromise as it controls for multiple comparisons without being too conservative
Sensitivity	Ability of a test to correctly identify the people with the condition under question. Sensitivity = true positive/(true positive + false negative)
Sensitivity analysis	A statistical technique used to examine uncertainties about a study's conclusions. Examples include one-way sensitivity analysis, extreme scenario analysis and Monte Carlo sensitivity analysis
Skewness	A departure from the normal distribution where either the 'left' or the 'right' hand tail of the distribution is longer than would be expected. **Positive skew:** The right hand tail is longer and the relationship between measures of central tendency is: mode <

median < mean. **Negative skew:** The left hand tail is longer and the relation between measures of central tendency is: mean < median < mode

Spearman's rank correlation	A non-parametric test, conventionally represented by the symbol r_s to distinguish it from correlation coefficient r. It uses differences between pairs of ranks rather than quantitative data similar to the parametric equivalent of correlation coefficient. It has the range: $-1 \leq r_s \leq 1$
Specificity	Ability of a test to correctly identify the people without the condition under question. Specificity = true negative/(true negative + false positive)
Standard deviation (SD)	A standardized measure of data dispersion based on deviations from the arithmetic mean
Standard error (SE)	A measure of uncertainty or dispersion, of a point estimate such as the sample mean. It is used to construct confidence intervals and is calculated as: $SD/\sqrt{n}$
Standardized mortality ratio	(Observed deaths/expected deaths) $\times$ 100
Stratification	Categorization of patients into groups defined by one or more important variables affecting outcome. This can be decided before randomization (pre-stratification) or at the time of analysis when the actual baseline variables affecting prognosis will be known (post-stratification)
Survival analysis	Aims to model the survival experience of individuals and to estimate associated quantities of interest. It is useful when the outcome is timed to an event. It assumes that dropouts have the same prognosis as those remaining in the study. The methods of data analysis include the log rank test and Cox's proportional hazards regression model. A Kaplan–Meier curve illustrates survival data
Survival curve	The horizontal sections indicate no change in the estimated probability for developing a disorder over a given period of time. The

vertical sections represent one or more patients developing a disorder. A sudden change in the estimated probability corresponds to times when an event, i.e. a disorder has occurred

t distribution

An important continuous probability distribution which, like the normal distribution, is symmetrical about the mean, but has longer tails than the standard normal distribution

Transformation

A change in the scale of a measurement by a mathematical function such as square root, log and inverse. It is done so that the data are normally distributed and parametric tests can be used

Triangulation

A combination of two or more theories, data source, methods or investigators in one study of a single phenomenon. If identical conclusions are drawn by using different methods, this enhances validity

t test

A parametric test for the differences between means of two populations. **Paired *t* test:** one-tailed *t* test is used where only one outcome is possible and two-tailed *t* test is used where there are two possible outcomes

Type 1 error

The situation where the null hypothesis is true but is rejected by a statistical test. It can be minimized by using Bonferroni's method or assessing less number of variables

Type 2 error

The situation where the null hypothesis is false but is accepted by a statistical test. It can be minimized by increasing the sample size

Utility

A health state preference score

Validity

A term used to describe whether an instrument measures what it purports to measure. Types of validity are as follows: **Concurrent validity:** The comparison of the measure being tested with an external valid yard stick at the same time. **Content validity:** The instrument measures the entire domain of what is to be measured. It may be particularly relevant in psychiatry because there is considerable overlap between different types of measurement. **Criterion validity:** The ability of an instrument to yield the same results as another known test to be valid. Concurrent and predictive validity together are sometimes called as criterion validity. **Cross validity:** Validation of a measurement which has its criterion validity established for one sample and then is retested on another sample. **External validity:** How well a test measures what it is supposed to measure and identifies what it is supposed to identify. **Face validity:** It is not validity at all, but it refers to the subjective judgement whether the measurement in question appears on the surface to measure the feature in question. It is of relevance only when an instrument appears to have absolutely no connection to the variable being measured. **Incremental validity:** It is the term used to indicate whether the measurement is superior to other measurements in approaching true validity. **Internal validity:** In the context of a treatment difference, it refers to the extent to which that difference can be reasonably attributed to treatment assignment. **Predictive validity:** It is a relatively uncommon measurement. It determines the extent of agreement between a present measurement and one in the future

Variable

Something (a quantity or attribute) that varies between individuals or items. A dependent (outcome) variable is plotted on Y axis and an independent (predictor) is plotted on X axis. There are two main types of variables. **Categorical or qualitative,** and **Numerical or quantitative.** Categorical variables are as follows. **Binary variables:** include dichotomous responses, e.g. male/female, yes/no, etc. Chi-squared test is suitable for them. **Nominal variables:** Where number is assigned to a category but does not indicate order or magnitude. Chi-squared test is suitable for them. **Ordinal variables:** They can be ranked in order but no assumptions made about the magnitude of the difference between the ranks. Non-parametric analyses are suitable for them. Numerical variables are as follows. **Continuous variables:** They take any values including fractions, e.g. temperature, blood pressure, etc. **Discrete variables:** They take only integral values, e.g. number of children in a house, number of houses in a locality, etc.

Relative frequency of a variable	Proportion of the total frequency that corresponds to that variable
Cumulative frequency of a variable	Total frequency up to that particular value
Variance	A standardized measure of data dispersion, equal to the standard deviation squared
Wilcoxon's rank sum test	Uses two independent samples to compare two populations with respect mainly to location. The sizes of the samples do not necessarily have to be equal but they must be independent and random
Wilcoxon's signed rank test	Used to compare non-qualitative matched paired samples or two repeated measures from one sample which are not normally distributed
Yates' correction	It is a process of subtracting 0.5 from the numerator at each term in the chi-squared statistic for 2×2 tables prior to squaring the term.
z score	A data transformation calculated by subtracting the mean from every value and dividing by the standard deviation

FURTHER READING

General textbooks

Buckley P, Bird J, Harrison G, Prewette G (2004) *Examination Notes in Psychiatry*, 4th edn. London: Hodder Arnold.

Gelder M, Mayou R, Cowen P (2004) *Shorter Oxford Textbook of Psychiatry*, 4th edn. Oxford: Oxford University Press.

Gelder MG, Lopez-Ibor J Jr, Andreasen NC (2003) *New Oxford Textbook of Psychiatry*. Oxford: Oxford University Press.

Sadock BJ, Sadock VA (2005) *Kaplan and Sadock's Comprehensive Textbook of Psychiatry*, 7th edn. Philadelphia: Lippincott Williams & Wilkins.

Johnstone E, Lawrie S, Owens D, Sharpe MD (2004) *Companion to Psychiatric Studies*, 7th edn. London: Churchill Livingstone.

Puri BK, Hall AD (2004) *Revision Notes in Psychiatry*, 2nd edn. London: Hodder Arnold.

Paykel ES (1992) *Handbook of Affective Disorders*, 2nd edn. Edinburgh: Churchill Livingstone.

Thornicroft G, Szmukler G (2001) *Textbook of Community Psychiatry*. Oxford: Oxford University Press.

Basic sciences

Malhi G, Malhi S (2005) *Examination Notes in Psychiatry: Basic Sciences*, 2nd edn. London: Hodder Arnold

Morgan G, Butler S (1993) *Seminars in Basic Neurosciences*. London: Gaskell.

Puri BK, Tyrer P (1998) *Sciences Basic to Psychiatry*. 2nd edn. London: Churchill Livingstone.

Weller M *et al.* (1991) *The Scientific Basis of Psychiatry*. London: WB Saunders.

Child psychiatry

Goodman R, Scott S (2005) *Child Psychiatry*, 2nd edn. Oxford: Blackwell Publishers.

Goodyer I (2001) The depressed child and adolescent: developmental and clinical perspectives. 2nd edn. Cambridge: Cambridge University Press.

Govers S (2005) *Seminars in Child and Adolescent Psychiatry*, 2nd edn. London: Gaskell.

Rutter M, Taylor E, Hersov L, eds. (1995) *Child and Adolescent Psychiatry: Modern Approaches*. Oxford: Blackwell Scientific.

Classification

American Psychiatric Association (1994) *Diagnostic and Statistical Manual of Mental Disorders: DSM-IV*, 4th edn. Washington, DC: APA.

World Health Organization (1992) *The ICD-10 Classification of Mental and Behavioural Disorders: Clinical Descriptions and Diagnostic Guidelines.* World Health Organization, Geneva.

Critical review

Ajetunmobi O. (2002) *Making sense of critical appraisal.* London: Hodder Arnold.
Brown T, Wilkinson G (2005) *Critical Reviews in Psychiatry,* 3rd edn. London: Gaskell.
Crombie I (1996) *Pocket Guide to Critical Appraisal.* London: BMJ Books.
Greenhaugh T (2000) *How to read a paper: The Basics of Evidence Based Medicine,* 2nd edn. London: BMJ Books.
Lawrie SM, McIntosh AM, Rao S (2001) *Critical Appraisal for Psychiatry.* London: Churchill Livingstone.
Sackett D (2000) *Evidence Based Medicine: How to practice and teach EBM.* 2nd edn. London: Churchill Livingstone.
Siegel S (1998) *Nonparametric statistics.* Singapore: McGraw Hill.
Swinscow TDV, Campbell MJ (1996) *Statistics at square one.* London: BMJ Publishing Group.

Descriptive psychopathology

Hamilton M (1985) *Fish's Clinical Psychopathology: Signs and Symptoms in Psychiatry,* 2nd edn. Bristol: John Wright.
Sims A (2002) *Symptoms in Mind: An Introduction to Descriptive Psychopathology,* 3rd edn. London: Bailliere Tindall.

Dynamic psychopathology/psychoanalysis

Edelson M (1990) *Psychoanalysis: A Theory in Crisis.* Chicago: University of Chicago Press.

Forensic psychiatry

Chiswick D, Cope R, eds. (1995) *Seminars in Practical Forensic Psychiatry.* London: Gaskell.
Gunn J, Taylor P (1994) *Forensic Psychiatry: Clinical, Legal and Ethical Issues.* Oxford: Butterworth Heinemann.

General adult psychiatry

Stein G, Wilkinson G (1998) *Seminars in General Adult Psychiatry.* Vols 1 and 2. London: Gaskell.

Learning disability

Fraser W, Kerr M (2003) *Seminars in Psychiatry of Learning Disability,* 2nd edn. London: Gaskell.

Liaison psychiatry

Guthrie E, Creed F (1996) *Seminars in Liaison Psychiatry.* London: Gaskell.

Mental health law

Jones R (2004) *Mental Health Act Manual*, 9th edn. London: Sweet and Maxwell Ltd.

Puri BK, Brown RA, Mckee HJ, Treasaden IH (2005) *Mental Health Law: A Practical Guide.* London: Hodder Arnold.

Miscellaneous

Department of Health (1999) *Code of Practice: Mental Health Act 1983.* London: HMSO.

Freeman H (1998) *Seminars in Psychosexual Disorders.* London: Gaskell.

McGuffin *et al.* (1994) *Seminars in Psychiatric Genetics.* London: Gaskell.

Old age psychiatry/organic psychiatry

Butler R, Pitt B (1998) *Seminars in Old Age Psychiatry.* London: Gaskell.

Lishman WA (1998) *Organic Psychiatry: The Psychological Consequences of Cerebral Disorder*, 3rd edn. Oxford: Blackwell Scientific.

Jacoby R, Oppenheimer C, eds (2002) *Psychiatry in the Elderly*, 3rd edn. Oxford: Oxford Medical Publications.

Psychology

Colman AM (2003) *Oxford Dictionary of Psychology.* Oxford: Oxford University Press.

Gupta D, Gupta R, eds (2003) *Psychology for Psychiatrists.* London: Whurr Publishers.

Munafo M (2002) *Psychology for the MRCPsych.* 2nd edn. London: Hodder Arnold.

Smith EE, Nolen-Hoeksema S, Fredrickson B, Loftus G (2003) Atkinson and Hilgard's Introduction to Psychology. 14th edn. USA: Wadsworth.

Tantam D, Birchwood M (1994) *Seminars in Psychology and Social Sciences.* London: Gaskell.

Psychopharmacology

Anderson IM, Reid IC (2004) *Fundamentals of Clinical Psychopharmacology*, 2nd edn. London: Taylor and Francis.

Bazire S (2005) *Psychotropic Drug Directory: The Professionals Pocket. Handbook and Aide Memoirè.* Philadelphia: Lippincott, Williams & Wilkins.

Cookson J, Taylor D, Katona C (2002) *Use of Drugs in Psychiatry*, 5th edn. London: Gaskell.

King D, ed. (2004) *Seminars in Clinical Psychopharmacology*, 2nd edn. London: Gaskell.

Mehta DK, ed. (2005) *British National Formulary.* Oxon: Pharmaceutical Press.

Stahl S (2000) *Essential Psychopharmacology: Neuroscientific Basis and Practical Applications*, 2nd edn. Cambridge: Cambridge University Press.

Taylor D, Paton C, Kerwin R. (2005) *The Maudsley 2005–2006 Prescribing Guidelines*, 8th edn. London: Taylor and Francis.

Psychotherapy

Bateman A, Holmes J (2000) *Introduction to Psychotherapy: An Outline of Psychodynamic Principles and Practice*, 3rd edn. London: Routledge.
Greenberger D, Padesky C (1995) *Clinician's Guide to Mind Over Mood*. New York: Guilford Press.
Hawton K, Salkovskis PM, Kirk J, Clark DM, eds (2000) Cognitive–behavioural approaches for adult psychiatric disorders: a practical guide. 2nd edn. Oxford: Oxford University Press.

Substance misuse

Chick J, Cantwell R, eds. (1994) *Seminars in Alcohol and Drug Misuse*. London: Gaskell.
Ghodse H (2002) *Drugs and Addictive Behaviour: A Guide to Treatment*, 3rd edn. Cambridge: Cambridge University Press.

Transcultural psychiatry

Bhugra D, Cochrane R (2001) *Psychiatry in Multicultural Britain*. London: Gaskell.

INDEX

Note: References for ISQs are given in the form of the starting page number followed in curled brackets by the question number(s) which may runover on to the following page(s). References for EMIs are distinguished from the ISQs by use of square brackets. References to all other sections have standard page numbering. A few indexed topics are mentioned just in the answer.